THE RED THREAD

Healing Possession at a Muslim Shrine in North India

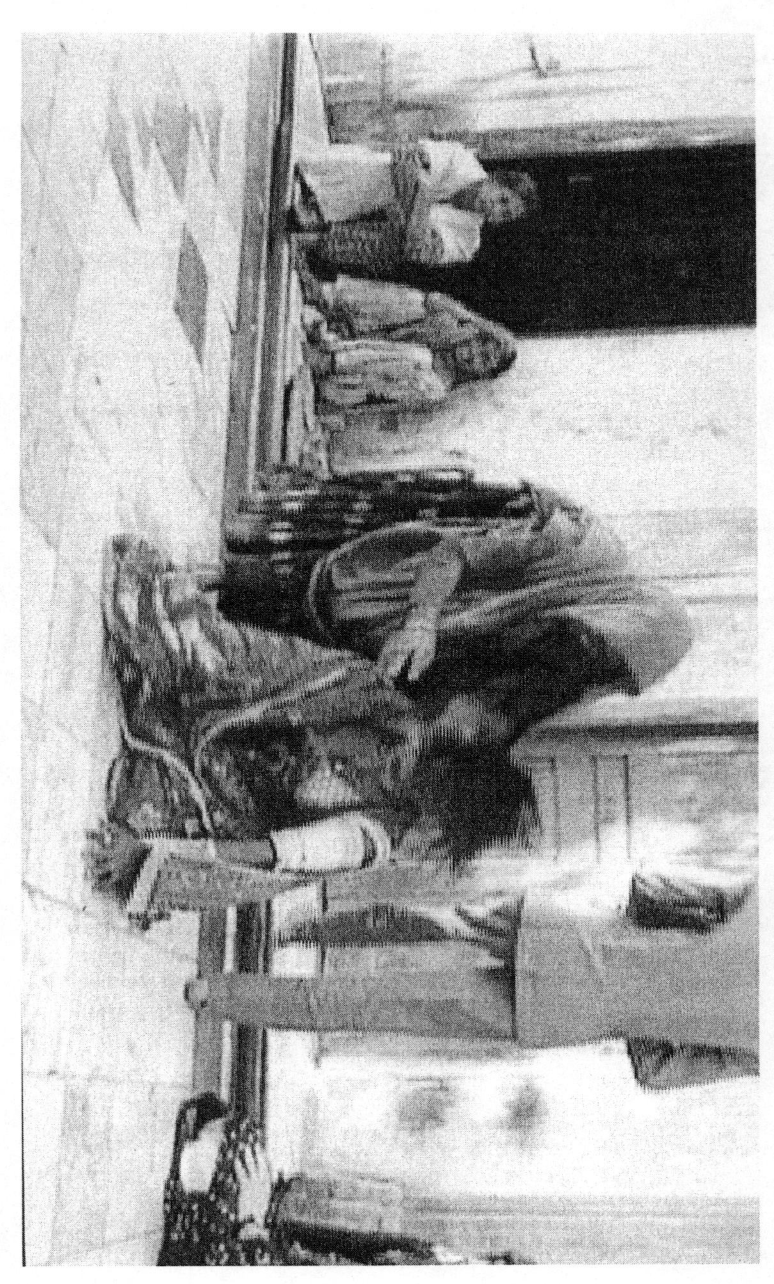

THE RED THREAD

Healing Possession at a Muslim Shrine in North India

Beatrix Pfleiderer

Translated from the German by Malcolm R. Green

Under Collaboration of Virchand Dharamsey

THE RED THREAD

First published as
Die besessenen Frauen von Mira Datar Dargah, Heilen und Trance in Indien
by
Campus Verlag GmbH, Frankfurt/Main, 1994

First Published, 2006

ISBN 81-87879-63-7

Published by
AAKAR BOOKS
28 E Pocket IV, Mayur Vihar Phase I, Delhi-110 091
Phone : 011-2279 5505 Telefax : 011-2279 5641
aakarbooks@bol.net.in; www.aakarbooks.com

Printed at
D.K Fine Art Press (P) Ltd., Delhi

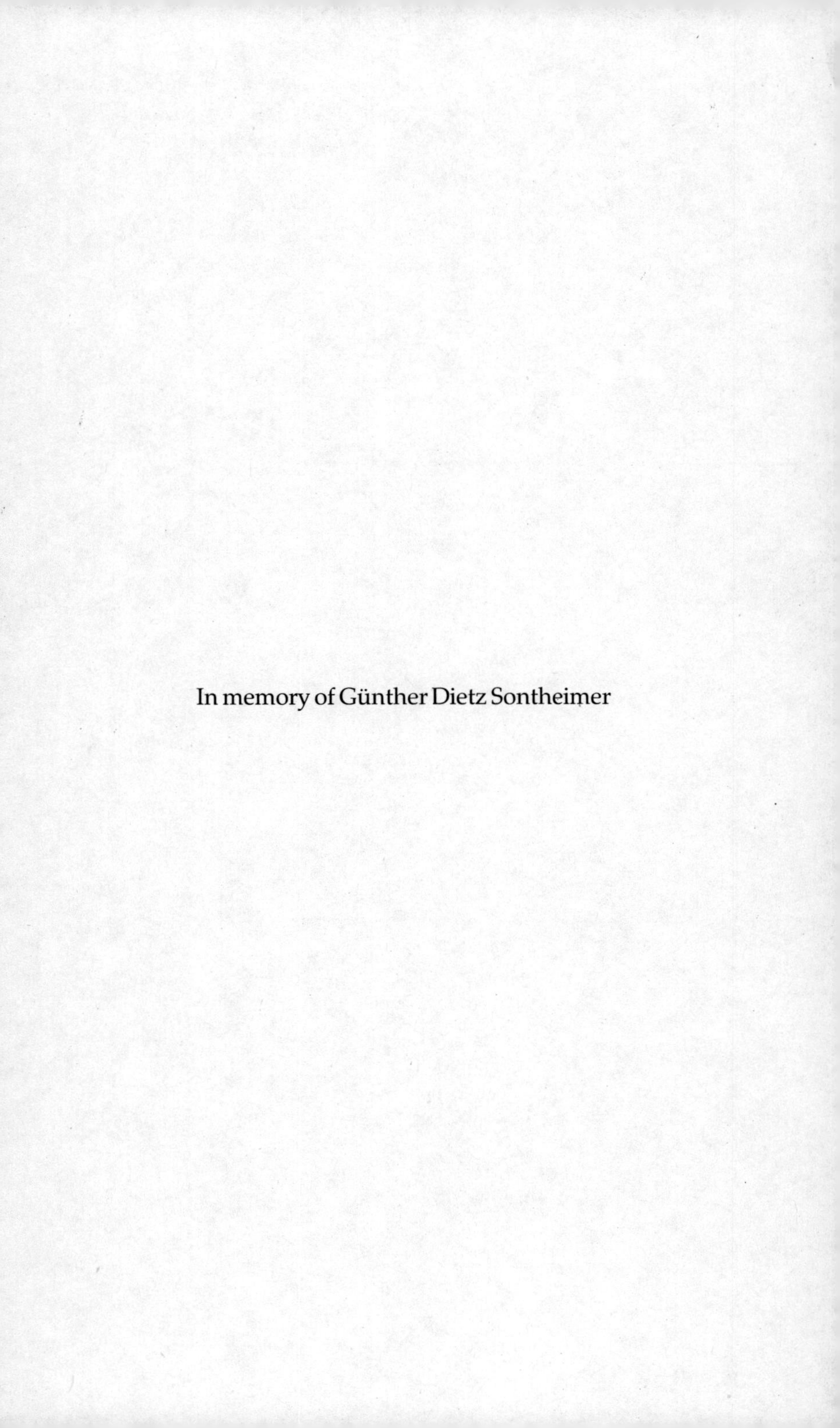

In memory of Günther Dietz Sontheimer

Contents

Foreword

The ethnographic studies which went to make up this book were conducted over ten years ago. My first visit to Unava was fifteen years ago, but the procedures at the Mira Datar tomb have remain unchanged, as I confirmed during my last visit in January 1992. The roles, the players and the play still have the same structural quality. All that has changed are the people who play the parts. A young fourteen year-old woman who apparently was possessed by the devil, and who last January raged about the inner court of the tomb, had not even been born when we commenced our studies. The possessed women have seen one generation follow on from another. It is now their daughters' turn to let the demons talk, rage and scream on the stage of Mira Datar's *dargah.* Even the guardians of the shrine, the *mujawars*, have witnessed the succession of generations. Muhammadhusen, the *Sajjadanashin* or highest dignitary, has died. His successor has not yet been designated.

And I, too, have "passed through a generation" between the ethnographic work on the tomb and the writing of this book. During my ten years as professor at the Institute of Anthropology at the University of Hamburg, I was able to supervise twenty-five doctoral candidates who worked on topics related to this book and confer on them their doctorates. What they don't realise is that everything I have drawn on for the work on this text I learned from them while aiding them in the process of writing their dissertations. They were my school, which is why I would like to thank them in this foreword.

During the years of my investigations a large number of discussions helped me to clarify and sort out the complicated social structure I wished to study there. My thanks go to Paul and Goldy Parin for the ethno-psychoanalytic eye they cast on the initial chaos of my data. I would also like to thank the anthropology students and psychotherapists who visited me in Unava and gave me their help, their company and their advice. Similarly my thanks go to all the travellers I was friends with, and who literally went out of their way to discuss with me some detail or other of the therapeutic process at the tomb. But most of all I would like to thank Lothar Lutze who, as a passionate expert on Indian culture and my companion during these years, also went out of his way on several occasions in order to visit the possessed women at the tomb and its administrators.

In 1980 the German Research Council funded my journey to visit traditional healers in north India and in 1981 supported me for eighteen months so that I could analyse the material on this topic at the Institute for Tropical Hygiene at the University of Heidelberg, a period I used to produce anthropology publications. I would like to acknowledge here the assistance I received from both these institutions.

My greatest thanks go however to Virchand Dharamsey who, as initially my translator and later my untiring co-researcher, conducted interviews at the tomb, located files and sources with the intention of gaining information on the economics and history of the shrine, and who, as billeting officer, contact maker, travel organiser and discussion partner, became a major part of this project. It would have been no fun without him. Although I have put Virchand Dharamsey on the title page on account of his tireless collaboration, I should point out here that I alone am responsible for the text of this book.

My colleague and friend Jyotindra Jain, director of the Crafts Museum in New Delhi, told me so much about Gujarat, possession, gods and goddesses, temples and trances during our time together as "post-doc" fellows at the South Asia Institute at Heidelberg University that I had no option but to travel there. I thank him for opening up Indian ethnography to me, for putting me hot on the tracks of the Mira Datar Dargah, and for revealing to me many other "shamanic" contexts in Gujarat and Rajasthan. I also thank him and his wife, Jutta Jain, for keeping the door of their house constantly open to Virchand Dharamsey, myself and our numerous visitors, and for the fact that we never as much as changed trains in Ahmedabad without first enjoying their hospitality. And finally I thank my friend, the painter Sarita Golani from Mumbai, who assisted me in many of the ethnographic studies I performed over the years in India and Sri Lanka. She worked at the tomb with the women and showed them how to paint what they experienced in trance.

I call this book an ethnographic narrative. It is focussed every bit as much on the process at the back of an ethnography and its basic impossibility, as on the many small incidents that arose each day and our attempts to deal with them. Since I attach importance to just such incidents in this text, all who were involved with me there will become actors, myself included. For this reason I do not wish to divulge their names. Consequently none of the names in this book are the actors' real names. This applies to everyone: to my visitors at my research site, to the *mujawars,* and to the pilgrims at the tomb. The sole exception is the *Sajjadanashin* Muhammadhusen, whose position in any case makes him a historic personality. I am grateful to him for our discussions and hope that I have portrayed them in a way that does him justice. The only other person in this ethnographic game whose identity has not been concealed is myself. And that is rightly so because I have to bear the responsibility for the staging and the text.

This book is dedicated to the memory of Günther Sontheimer, a friend who generously allowed me and a good many others to participate in his studies of possession cults in Maharashtra and thus taught us to read India.

Kalapana, Hawai'i, B.P.
May 1993

Preface : Two fables

The Cunning Wife

There once was a parrot. And he had a wife. One day the parrot felt the desire to eat milk rice. The parrot said to his wife: "Hey, wife, make me some milk rice!" The female parrot replied: "I haven't any rice, haven't any sugar, and haven't any milk either — so how am I to make milk rice for you!" The parrot quickly went and fetched rice, sugar and milk, and his parrot wife made milk rice for him. After she had made the milk rice she said to her husband: "It's time you went for a wash!" The parrot went for a wash — and while he was away the female parrot ate up all the milk rice and flew off. That's the end of story. It was nothing more than that.

Told by Banubai from Karaj, Mithila/Bihar

The Guileless Girl

A boy and a girl fell in love. They attended the same college. And their bodies also loved each other, so they remained together once they had completed their time at college. One day the girl's family received an offer of marriage from a well-to-do family. She was to marry the family's son, who was a doctor. Her lover came from simpler circumstances and worked in the building trade. She hurried to him and said: "I am going to get engaged to a doctor and marry him. As for us, nothing will change, we shall remain lovers." He replied: "That is not possible. You must decide on one of us. And if you marry someone else there is no more reason for me to carry on living in this world." The girl thought to herself: that is what he says now, but later he will get used to it, and she went and married the doctor. On the day of the wedding her lover hung himself.

When the wedding night came she told her husband that it was the wrong time of the month, and with that their first night passed by. The following day she went to back to her parent's home because she was seized by inexplicable anxiety. She was told that her lover had taken his life on the day of the wedding. She had not reckoned with anything like that.

She returned to her husband. He had been knocked over by something invisible as it had grown dark. "Are you drunk?" the woman asked. "No," the man replied, "I felt an obstacle that barred my way, and then I fell over." The woman's anxiety grew and turned into an illness. Her husband could not help her, and nor could any of the other doctors. She was taken to the grave of a Muslim saint, Mira Datar. Her husband found out about her story as she began talking there with the voice of her lover. Her lover told her that he would not allow her to have any physical relations with her husband. The husband and the girl annulled their marriage. So now she has no one, neither the one nor the other. And no one can have her any more.

Told by a *mujawar* at the inner court of Mira Datar Dargah.

Chapter 1

Introduction

Every book, or every work that aspires to become one, is triggered by something inexplicable, something that suddenly enters a person's life without plan and without even a place for it. That's how it was for me, at least. The leaflet that set this book rolling was lying on the cobbles of the courtyard in the rain. I was just on my way to hold a lecture as part of the course I was giving at the University of Hawaii in Hilo during the academic year 1990–1991. And there on the ground I saw a leaflet which said: "Experience the world of trance through the wisdom of your breath!" It intrigued me. I picked up the leaflet, which gave more information about the wheres and whens and how long one had to allow oneself to be lured away from everyday life. I decided to give it a go and dialled the number. A woman answered and gave me the worldly information that I had to enclose one hundred dollars with my enrollment form so that it would be valid, and that I should bring a blanket, a sleeping bag and comfy clothing. "And perhaps a blindfold," she added. "What on earth's that for?" I asked myself. I turned up at the appointed time. The experience led me to a strange, remote place in a valley that was very reminiscent of the foothills of the Himalayas where, over ten years previously, I had studied the work of healers who enter into trance. I felt as though I was travelling to a familiar place. Some twenty people arrived for the archaic experience that had been announced, and now ascended the stairs to the practice room of this "retreat" with blankets and meditation cushions tucked under their arms. We all sat down in a circle. The workshop leaders talked about trance, shamans and transpersonal psychology. They also said that it is everyone's birthright to experience the rapture and ecstasy that one can experience through trance therapy. "What happens if you don't experience it?" one of the participants wanted to know, and another asked, slightly concerned, whether anything bad could happen, whether one could accidentally end up in demonic ecstasy instead of holy rapture. Our minds were put at rest. Whatever happened, we were told, would be exactly what we required at that moment. We were now instructed to lie down on our mats, close our eyes, direct our breathing inwards and deepen it. While the participants meekly obeyed the instructions, a pair of enormous loud speakers inundated the breathers with drumming music at top volume. The drum rhythms from African and Asian cultures were shortly followed by the more complex sound forms of New Age music. The way the music infiltrated the people's bodies was not without its effect. Some got up and began snake-like dances, others tossed back and forth as if in feverish delirium, while yet others roared like lions or sobbed like babes. It was as if all hell had broken loose, or some stupendous drug had been taken: everything had gone simply wild. Only when the long drawn-out sounds of a flute and calm string music flowed into the room did the madness abate. Calm was slowly restored, still broken though by sighs, laughs, muttering, prayers and the like—all the modes of expression that come when people are emotionally shaken.

As the music finished I went down the steps outside to the palms. The surrounding landscape seemed like the continuation of the journey from which I had just surfaced. The two workshop leaders had been right, the journey had brought me to an unknown rapture. My body was still flooded with the energy I had experienced there on my mat. I tried to recall what I had encountered on my inner journey. My notes from then tell the following:

> "I breathe. As deeply and intensely as possible. Just as I had resolved to do, and with that a beautiful meadow appears before me on which I want to stay a while. I breathe shallower, but the

> sitter's hand reminds me — it's breath-work! It's work! — and I go back to fast breathing. New music comes, from Africa. I see African dancers before me. I feel the energy of an African woman dancing, I feel myself in her body. The dancing energy becomes more and more my own. The music goes on. It carries the energy, it transports me. I breathe fast and deep, breathe more and even more. And all of a sudden it's there: I see the creation, or I am in the creation, or a part of it as it is brought into being by the dance. I dance and stamp and channel the energy down to where I create and create and dance and dance and stomp and stomp. And an enormous amount of energy comes into being. Everything is spinning, everything is chaos! And is coming into being: and then the earth comes into being!!! And I think the work is done. I enter another time. I enter out into space. And an enormous joy fills me, joy far beyond anything mortal, yes real joy. And more and more joy comes into being inside me, emanates from me. Joy, beautiful divine sparks. My body is full, full, full of energy. My body saw Shiva, my body was Shiva, knows his energy and radiates it, knows how it must stamp, everything was blue during Shiva's dance.
>
> Once the creation is complete I enter the water age. It is quiet. All that is there is a turtle. It swims and holds the creation together. Swims round and round, busily, solicitously encircling the earth. Which has now grown green and has the turtle as its mount."

I related my experience later to the group during the "exchange" session. "You've encountered an archetype," the group leaders said, "you have experienced the Indian creation myth." Still slightly perplexed and astonished, I went back to my car and drove down the valley to the coastal road that leads to Hilo.

And all the while I recalled the scenes that the possessed women in India stage with the same screams, dances, convulsions and moans that I had heard today: the women I encountered at the tomb of the Muslim saint in north-west India, and whose voices I recorded a good ten years ago on film and tape. I had asked them to tell me about the images and journeys they experienced in trance, and now I saw them again in front of me, kneeling in the courtyard and breathing fast. Before my inner eye I could see the stage of these women on which I, too, worked for many months as an anthropologist. Although I had dutifully brought everything that they had told me to the public eye in anthropological publications, the finished text was so deeply encoded that it was unable to affect anyone in the way that was demanded by what I had heard and seen. "I must write a book about the stage of the women in trance, an entire book just about that," I thought, "and straight away!" Two weeks later I had begun work.

I had to write the book because the way trance was dealt with publicly at this tomb was not that dissimilar to the way trance was dealt with in the workshop I had just attended. There were unmistakable parallels. And the more people there are in the West who wish to experience trance for reasons of therapy or self-discovery, the more important I feel it is to describe the same activity in other cultures. We need to know how others tackle it, what the setting is like, as well as the mental set in which the trance is evoked and used for healing psychic wounds. So I dug out my carefully hoarded ethnographical material, took it out of its cardboard boxes, listened to the tapes and read through the notebooks. Shortly after, I began writing this book.

It describes the ethnographic path I took to discover the procedures and occurrences at a Muslim shrine (or monumental tomb) in the north of the Indian state of Gujarat. The tomb lies to the north of the district town of Mehsana in a small village named Unava, close to Unjha railway station. In spring one can see piles of cumin seed, or *jeera* in Hindustani, that reached to the rafters; the aroma is inseparable for me from my ethnographical work there. When mixed with water, *jeera* acts as a cooling medicine during hot weather. But if too much is taken the body displays signs of overheating. What that means is shown in turn by the stories that are told at the Mira Datar Dargah.

In both the ethnographic literature as well as in Indian officialese, the term Muslim shrine stands for a Muslim centre of pilgrimage or tomb. In this book I shall mainly use the word tomb, even though it distracts attention from the fact that the shrine consists of numerous tombs. Muslim shrines are tombs which house the mortal remains of a *pir*, a Muslim saint (and often his relatives and pupils as well) who has performed miracles. This is also the reason why the people who visit his grave assume it still has the power to perform miracles, *karamat* in Hindustani. These tombs can be found all over India in places where Muslims have lived. Sometimes they consist solely of a white stone surround and a memorial slab, surmounted by a green flag proclaiming the doings of Islam, and an inscription giving the name of the *pir* who rests there. At other times they are large sites that cover whole sections of towns, such as the shrine of the Sufi mystic Mu'in al-din Chishti in Ajmer. In Hindustani, the lingua franca of northern India, Muslim shrines are termed *dargah*, which means approximately court or even royal court. I have described their origins in Sufiism in Chapter IV, "The tomb and its order". The tomb as such is Muslim but, as will be seen in this chapter, the visitors come from every class, creed, caste and region of India. The tomb is consequently a matter of pan-Indian importance. I have also described our arrival there in the same chapter.

Everything that I have recorded in this book I learned during my conversations with the people who do what I shall describe here. At the beginning I lacked a secure grasp of the language in which we conducted out conversations and required the assistance of an interpreter. We made our first trip to "our" *dargah* in 1977, while drawing up our plans for the study. The work proper began in 1980 and continued, with interruptions, until 1982. By the time I no longer wished to have an interpreter between me and my opposite number, he had become so familiar with the day-to-day life and running of the *dargah* that he continued to conduct the study with me until its completion. He generally spoke with the guardians of the tomb, the *mujawars*, while I mostly spoke with the women who had come to the *dargah* because they were possessed by demons. I have reported all that we were able to learn about the shrine in Chapters V and VI. Chapter V describes the possessed women on their stage, which I have later described as "without a history" in the seventh and final chapter. Chapter VI talks about the institution, which amounts to the history of the men.

This book also describes my first journey across India in the chapter entitled "The journey, the question and the field". This journey was not long, perhaps two weeks in all. Nevertheless it was endless because it engendered all the subsequent journeys that I made in India in compliance with the "question" of possession that was on my mind, and which I have interspersed in my text — which makes it so confusing, just as initially India was confusing to me. Only from Chapter IV onwards will the text will start to gain in clarity, when it focuses on the ethnography of trance and possession.

The first journey took me just from Mumbai (former Bombay) to Unava in Gujarat, to the "field" that is described in this book. We, the interpreter and I, travelled by rail, in buses, on rickshaws, by foot and in the proverbial Indian ox-carts. We travelled by day and by night. And on our way we spoke with everyone we met about healers, spirit possession, gods and goddesses, temples and trance. And almost everyone helped us on our way, gave us the name of the next healer "by the wayside", took us to concealed temples through the labyrinthine backstreets of the old parts of town or pointed the way through the fields to the hut of some healer they knew. Or they invited us to eat, or put us up for the night — according to the time of day. The food they offered seemed like paradise to me. It was as if my childhood dreams had all come true, and all on the same day. Because everything they gave us to eat instantly became my favourite dish, regardless whether it was one of the famous and highly varied *thalis* from Gujarat, on which up to twenty different foods are served simultaneously, or a simple dish of rice and lentils made with such beguiling spices that it was fit for a palace. Never in my life have I felt so well looked after as in this land of seemingly perfect hospitality.

On one occasion, while we were wandering across the fields from one village to the next under the blistering midday sun, I found the heat so unbearable that I refused to budge from the feeble shade of a small bush. My interpreter carried on until he managed to obtain a beaker of water in a nearby hut and brought it back to me. This life-giving water in the sparkling metal container was all that I could have wished for at that moment. All that we experienced was for me a live performance of the *Thousand and One Nights*. And I knew at once that I never wanted to leave here again, and if I did have to I wanted to return as soon as possible in order to set out again along the paths of this dreamtime. This journey produced a great many fundamental changes in me and left me with a fascination for this culture from which I was never to be free.

India "is" one of the wisest and most magnificent cultures ever to come into being on this planet (with the qualification that the developments in this culture under the influence of modern Islam and colonialism have robbed woman of much of her former space). Perhaps I would not be able to admit my fondness for an entire culture quite so freely here if one of my first diaries had not contained this very sentence, albeit written in a foreign hand. The great Indian scholar A.L.Basham wrote it for me among my notes, with the additional remark: "and the greatest form of entertainment that exists is the Indian film". That was a trail that I had no intention of leaving.

Since the path I was pursuing at home was that of a scientific career, I applied to the German Research Council for funding to enable me to conduct one study on traditional healers, and another on the Hindi movie — which is also a universal palliative in India. My applications were granted and I was given the freedom and possibility to make repeated visits, on one occasion for a whole eighteen months.

When however the continuation of "my personal Indian dreamtime" brought me into the hot months preceding the monsoon, during which one can no longer walk unprotected in the sun and the earth in the fields grows cracked and infertile under its parching rays, my *Thousand and One Nights* started to look a little frayed at the edges and I began to value the return ticket I had stashed away in my luggage. On one occasion, while waiting for a taxi outside of my hotel before taking my return flight from Mumbai, I was approached by a woman wearing a European style dress, an unusual thing in the land of the sari, so evidently she was an Anglo-Indian, who asked me: "Where do you go?" I answered: "I'll fly back to Germany", to which she replied, "Lucky girl." This encounter occupied my thoughts for a long while, and in many ways rectified the views I had held during my initial "honeymoon" period. I have never forgotten the woman and was reminded of her while working on the "case" of the DeSilva family (see Chapter V, "The curse, the spirits and their magicians").

This book also describes a different approach, a different path than the normal mental and physical considerations of ethnography. The pursuit of this path runs all the way through the chapters of this book: it is the attempt to understand trance and possession. While Chapter III merely reports on the helplessness, the search and the astonishment at a phenomenon that has been removed from our European field of vision, Chapters IV and V focus on what the women told me about the way they handle possession and trance. I relate what they say while they are *inside* trance, in what they call *hajri*, which roughly means in the presence of the demon or demoness. This text, which is intended to explain how the women deal with *hajri*, has often been left in the form of the original dialogues. It is these dialogues, which are part and parcel of finding out about trance and other states of consciousness, that are what are commonly termed "extraordinary". At the same time I shall report on spaces, above all in Chapter V, but also from an evaluative standpoint in Chapter VII — spaces which women can open up for themselves by means of possession within the restrictions imposed on them by their culture.

In Chapter VII I also summarise and recall our own history of possession, of out-of-the-ordinary states of consciousness among women, while recalling that I was unable to call this to mind while talking with the women at the tomb. So in this final chapter I catch up with a small historical digression that had been missing from my baggage while I was playing the anthropologist.

This book is above all a treatise on women. The meaning

of the German title *The Possessed Women of Mira Datar Dargah* faithfully depicts the content and inner sequence of the questions I examined. It is about possession and the stage, the *dargah*, on which the possession is acted out. The players are the women and the stage, the *dargah*, is secondary. The *dargah* provides the props, the space, the surface which they have occupied, and thus also clamours to be described (Chapter VI).

The first time I saw the *dargah* I knew that here answers could be found to the "questions" that I had brought with me. Because possession, the idiom of possession, is simply the possibility of annexing space by means of cunning. And that is what the women do here. With possession they choose a means of expression that is incompatible with their everyday role. They set out on new paths inasmuch as they make what can be termed the "hidden discourse" their own; they talk with a language that cannot and must not have anything official about it. With that they create an incredibly effective possibility for themselves — acoustically, socially and psychologically — because here they can scream out the unspeakable. And this possibility will be described here.

The Indian woman has to be very cunning because she lives in a two-fold patriarchy, the Indian and the colonial. She relies on her cunning for the strength that every Western visitor is struck by, and which allows her to be the *devi*, the goddess, of the household. And this is what Banu, the mother of Ramnath Kumar from Mithila in the state of Bihar illustrated to me in her tale of the female parrot. "Go and have a wash, husband," the wife says, and with that she constrains her husband to comply with society's rules. Only once he has gone does she cook her pot of rice and eat it up. She creates the space for her actions by reminding her husband of the rules of Hindu social theory and thus binding him to them. This space offers a measure of freedom to her which she seizes, *for she really does fly away while he goes and has a wash*. The *women at the tomb also fly away* by liberating themselves from the rules that surround their bodies. And they likewise liberate themselves from the regulations on speech. They deviate from the course of submission by assuming the speech of the demons, just as an actress puts on a mask, the persona, in order to transform her existence. And it is this transformation that helps them against the programmatic excision of their egos that culture lays down for them.

For this reason I considered it necessary to describe the Hindu social theory of woman in Chapter II, so that the reader will understand the space in which women move inside the traditional Indian culture. Hopefully the space from which they come when they seize the idiom of possession and use the stage of the *dargah* to act out their own private myths will become sufficiently familiar to readers in Chapter II to give them the necessary perspective for reading the subsequent chapters. Chapter II is in fact a report on the existing literature. But I have also included scenes from the conversations I conducted with the women of a mountain village in northern India in 1980 and 1986. In addition I visited Banu, the mother of my research assistant for my project on the Indian film, Ramnath Kumar, in her village. Here I came to learn about the drastic succession of generations within one life: daughter — wife — mother-in-law — widow, and the often traumatic changes in identity that this brings about. And there I also learned about the cunning of the women and with that the she-parrot that speaks for the women in the fable on the first page of this book. The women of the village in Mithila instructed me in the topography of the paths that lead to the necessary cunning that allows them to survive.

But the men's stage, which I term the stage of order, also makes up part of my book on women. Chapter VI, which is concerned with the ethnography of Muslim shrines, describes the activities of the administrators, their life and their function. But it also tells of the men who come to this stage when their world has been shattered under the sheer weight of their lives and for whom the shrine offers a space for refuge. In this chapter we hear how men talk about women. Their conversations assign woman the space from which she attempts to liberate herself on the stage of the shrine during her *hajri* play. In this talk woman is artless, a person who must simply adhere to the rules. This is the woman whom the shrine attendants, the *mujawars*, talk about.

The fable of the young girl and her lover who hung himself and turned into a demon that speaks from her, tells of the women's hopelessness. The message here is: order or death, and it admits no cunning. "So now she has no one, neither the one nor the other. And no one can have her any more," says the *mujawar*, who keeps quiet about the cunning side of women that he fears while talking to me.

Chapter 2

The Cunning Women

> Never, no never put menstrual blood in your husband's food or else he will go mad, is bound to go mad.
>
> (A young woman in the court of the Mira Datar tomb)

When Phulan Devi, the bandit queen, divested her body of its weapons in February 1983 before the garlanded pictures of Gandhi and the benevolent goddess Durga, as well as before thousands of witnesses, and placed them of her own free will before these self-same pictures in an act of surrender, she gained enormous attention from the Indian and Western press (Sen,1991). An Indian woman in the form of a bandit queen, who is reputed to have set out from her countless hiding places in the Chambal Valley, the legendary "valley of the bandits", and mowed down over eighty cops? That does not fit the picture of either a Hindu or a Muslim woman. Yet Phulan Devi's fate and actions are perfectly logical when one remembers the hopeless situation into which she was born. After being married off by her parents at eleven, her parents-in-law sent the weak, sickly child-woman, who had known nothing but exploitation from an early age, back to her parental home with the demand for more dowry, only to be received by her mother with the words: "It would be better for you if you were dead," because there, too, order was more important than life. She shot open a space for herself "with a shooter" and maintained it over the years as the leader of her gang. She chose one of many possible strategies for expanding her field of action. Perhaps even Phulan Devi had visited a *dargah* on one or more occasions in order to scream the demons away from her body. Despite her unusual career, she was a "typical Indian" woman. And the signs of wisdom during her ritual surrender — before Gandhi, the socially acceptable revolutionary, before Durga, the deity who for all her goodness teaches men the meaning of fear — had its effect on her pursuers: the bandit is still alive, even if it meant she landed up in gaol: swapped spaces?

When Indian tree-felling firms were on the point of destroying the environment and life worlds of the women in Kumaun and Garhwal in the foothills of the Himalayas, the women hugged the threatened trees and remained so until the lumberjacks departed. With that they were able to retain lasting possession of their vital source of energy — the trees, whose twigs and leaves they use to feed their animals and fuel their stoves — and to found and maintain India's first ecology movement, which later was to spread to other regions of the country. In addition numerous farmers', smallholders' and agricultural workers' movements were launched and sustained by women, by poor farming women, in order to protect themselves against increasing impoverishment and growing exploitation. In her extensive study on the situation of Indian women, Maria Mies shows, how time and again it was women who gave the decisive push to mobilise the people during the "farmers' uprisings". Mies also reports on the feminist woman in this study, Indische Frauen zwischen Unterdrückung und Befreiung [= Indian women between suppression and liberation] (1985), and on the emergence of women from marriage under the old Indian patriarchy into independence and professional working life.

Although Indian women live in a "two-fold patriarchy", as I will mention several times in this book, it differs little from that of the West. The difference is primarily one of emphasis. While the majority of Indian women are married off by their parents and are ritually and economically dependent on their husbands, women in the occupational groups of India's upper social strata have better cards than us in the West, where, for instance, only six per cent of university lecturers are women, and the situation is much the same for, among others, gynaecologists. The Hindu woman Indira Gandhi, who was of the noblest Brahmin blood, was one of the most powerful women in the world, and her colleague in neighbouring Pakistan, Benazir Bhutto, was presumably the first female Muslim head of state. Admittedly the space occupied by these two professional politicians was inherited from their fathers, but it was they themselves who conquered and secured it — in female fashion.

This book is not concerned with "the Indian woman". She does not exist. The diversity is too large, too overwhelming for that. I am concerned here with describing strategies for coping, and have selected one of them as the topic of this book: spirit possession. Every woman from every social stratum, caste and religion is free to choose spirit possession as a means of expressing her psychic and social dis-ease. Those who have selected this route will have their say — in the *dargah* and here in this book.

Consequently this chapter is to be thought of as a lexicon — a lexicon of behaviour patterns which are derived from the old Indian patriarchy and which mould the notions about women that are brought up in this book. This chapter is concerned then with the basic assumptions of men and women about woman's existence. The later chapters, which report solely on the possessed women at the tomb, can be read in the light of these underlying assumptions. What I shall be writing about in this chapter is the general, commonplace knowledge about women in India. I shall draw on data from the cited literature and from field research I performed in a Himalayan mountain village in Uttar Pradesh, where for several years I interviewed women on their lives. These women live in the Hindu tradition and practise the Hindu social theory in an everyday manner, just as is written down in such classic ancient Indian texts as the *Dharmashastra*. What I wanted to discover and report on through the conversations I held at the village and later at the Muslim tomb was precisely this Hindu theory of woman in its daily practice.

Present-day Hinduism and modern Islam are two cultural systems that have reduced woman's space to such an extent that there is practically nothing left for her to live in. The Indian woman is assigned in every phase of her life to a man who has total power over her: her father, her husband and, after his death, her son. She brings from her father a highly elaborate ritual of surrender to her husband: marriage or *shadi*, which is a central topic in Hindu India. This transaction plunges the two families involved into a prolonged state of turmoil, for it is important to ensure that one has the right place in society so that one's daughter can be transferred to a sufficiently high social position. The daughter in this transaction is a means to an end. And remains so, for her duty in the new family is to guarantee the continuation of the line. In my opinion the view on the interdependency of the partners in marriage that is forwarded in the uncommonly large body of literature on the Indian woman is too one-sided. The dependency is two-fold, even if the visible data (the husband may remarry at any time if his wife does not outlive the marriage, whereas the woman may not) suggests at first sight a very one-sided dependency. I for my part think that the wife who finds her possibilities being "reduced" in such an extreme way by the Hindu and Muslim patriarchies is well aware of a number of strategies that will create space for her. Such spaces can help her to survive inside the patriarchal straitjacket. These thoughts are expressed in the following text from a Tamil epic, in which the woman's chastity is rewarded with the flame:

> Then I
> shall be a
> chaste woman
> when the flame
> lays hold to
> the wood.
>
> Then
> I shall be a noble woman
> when the fire cooks
> the gruel for the bellies

of my children.

As the chaste woman spoke this,
the flame flickered up
from the logs
until it reached the pot.

From the Tamil epic *Natalatankal*

I want to examine two of these spaces in the present book: the stage at Mira Datar's tomb, as a physical space, and trance, as a mental space. These are the two spaces that I shared and discussed with the women for a number of years. They are also spaces on which little has been written or could be read to date. I would like to refer to the women's life and actions in these "unofficial" spaces as the hidden discourse.

But first of all I would like to say something *about* the knowledge *about* Indian women that has accumulated outside of India, as well as about the images of the Indian woman that are conveyed to us by the press, literature, ethnography and Indology. This conventional knowledge about Indian women has been brought together in this chapter as a kind of lexicon so that it may form the basis for what is said later. For it is my belief that the normal manner of just presenting formal aspects has neglected the subtler images and the informal spaces and possibilities that are available to women. My main interest in this book is to portray such "unofficial" everyday practices and life strategies, and perhaps to add to what has already been written.

Seen from the outside, it is generally assumed, and quite rightfully, that the Indian woman is powerless and lacks any personal freedom of movement under both Hinduism and Islam. In principle the representatives of anthropology, as well as other observers, assume that the Indian woman remains throughout her life in the power or under the control of "the man" — in the shape of the father, the husband and the son. Other reports and studies endorse this initial observation. Inside the Indian Union there are some nine hundred women to a thousand men, while the reverse is true for the rest of the world. How has this come about?

This is explained in the medico-sociological literature, as well as in the grey, unpublished literature, by the fact that the introduction of amniocentesis (an examination of the amniotic fluid aimed at identifying genetically damaged foetuses, but which can also be misused solely to identify the child's sex) has led to the setting up of abortion clinics which even the poorest of the poor will visit. For five hundred rupees they can ensure that they will give birth to the son they so desire, while the unwanted daughter is not even given the chance to live. Some anthropologist friends of mine, who were working at the same time in the "neighbouring valley" in the Himalayas, added that: "In our village they don't even need amniocentesis to prevent female infants. The woman's mother-in-law places a grain of poison at the back of the newly-born girl's cheek two days after birth — all very discreetly and so that no one notices. That helps the mother, who then won't have to suckle the new-born baby over the years and can prepare herself for the next birth, which will hopefully be of the intended son".

Other press reports concerning the Indian family tell us that it is still assumed in Delhi that, in addition to the seven hundred dowry murders reported each year, there is an equal number of unreported cases. To which it should be added that the English had to abolish *sati* during the previous century because here once again women were being sacrificed. By whom? And for whom, one asks.

Dowry murders are a phenomenon of post-colonial India and are linked with the emergence of the middle classes and the creation of their property. In village life a woman leaves her family when she gets married. Her new family, her in-laws, get the benefit of her labour and her fertility. She becomes an economical asset for her new family. In town, however, the family is supported by a salary rather than by farming, so consequently a television, a car, a motorbike or a sofa set have to be extorted from the wife's family as an equivalent for the work that she no longer has to do in food production. As such the wife remains a means of production, though, on the road to the middle class world. Dowry murders are an urban phenomenon, where they are ubiquitous. *Sati*, which even today is occasionally forced upon women in more remote districts, had a different function: a woman was tied to her husband while he was alive, both ritually and economically, so it was only "logical" that she should not outlive him. I have the suspicion though that in this way the husband could protect himself from any evil designs on the part of his wife, for it is hard to equate *sati* with providing one's widow with a life assurance. Widows are no longer burned these days, but in traditional villages their hair is still shorn off. They become scarcely visible with their short layer of stubble hidden beneath their faded saris — or all too visible. Likewise their glass bangles are removed from them so that they can no longer be heard. And who indeed wants to hear them? They bring misfortune. Widows are not invited anywhere. They are a left-over, as the villagers say.

There are tooth goddesses and breast goddesses, writes Wendy D. O'Flaherty in her entertaining book *Women, Androgynes, and Other Mythical Beasts* (1980). Tooth goddesses decapitate, slay and otherwise kill their male companions, as is vividly portrayed by the praying mantis. (We also know the parallel concept of the *vagina dentata* from other cultures.) On the other hand, breast goddesses live a life of constant devotion and submission to their husbands. The former, the tooth goddess, is represented by Devi, the *Mahisa* who slays the buffalo demon as it approaches and courts her. The latter, the breast goddess, is represented by Sita, who remained all the time faithful to her husband Rama until, finally, his suspicions about her fidelity drove his despairing consort to leap into a crevice. Indian men can be heard saying (and sighing) *Sita jaise* (just like Sita) when they describe a woman who corresponds to the ideal of the breast goddess. Both types of women move, stimulate, feed (and kill) man. Both make him tremble: the one in awe, the other in fear and through her fruit, the son.

The notion that women in "patriarchal" Hindu India are controlled by men must be countered here by the idea that women themselves draw up *and* maintain the "game of the rules", which gives them the *appearance* of being under male control. And the idea that they subject men to their own control by assigning to them what seems sensible to assign to them. With this, women not only follow their mythical models, like the ones mentioned just now, but also implement what they in any case possess in the form of collective knowledge. This collective knowledge is, when it comes to the Hindu goddesses, closely connected with the collective unconscious. And this is fed by classical texts, just as it has similarly produced these texts. Let us take a look at the following connection in an old law book:

Manu, the son of the (male) sun *Surya*, who was the author of a lawbook (the *Dharmasastra*) and the first mortal, says: "Though he may have no good qualities or virtue, yet a husband must be constantly worshipped as a god by a faithful wife". To which Wendy O'Flaherty notes that the "Hindu lawbooks remind us *ad nauseam* that the Hindu wife [should] regard her husband as a god". (O'Flaherty, 1980, p.259) How long has this been the case, for it has a ring of "from one eternity to the next" about it? Might it be that the Aryan groups, those nomadic barbarians, had insufficient numbers of women with them and were thus put in the unpleasant position of having to accept the women of the sedentary peoples they had just subjugated? In northern India people still prefer to marry their daughters into higher social ranks. This custom is referred to as hypergamy, if one wanted to look it up in an anthropological dictionary. And daughters also always lead their married lives in the home of their parents-in-law, "in an alien world" as it were, for it is customary for them to leave their villages after the wedding. Although this "marrying above" leads to the daughters being respected as the future bearers of sons, it does not lead them to being treated as an equal to the son, who belongs to a higher-placed *jati* or local group. On marrying she leaves her lineage *(gotra)* and leaves her father's domain, as is underlined by numerous symbols. The wedding day is the day for the handing-over ceremony. The dowry is handed over. One piece after another, and each item undergoes careful inspection. In the foothills of the Himalayas, in the village of Gahar Banauliya where I lived with the women of the land-owner caste *(Kshatriya)*, it was anything but simple to see by night, without electric lighting, what the *larkilog* (the people from the bride's side) had packed into the chests. For which reason the groom's father demanded emphatically and without the slightest trace of humour that each item be removed from the chest and spread out on the floor, so that the number and quality of the items could be established. During this the village women sang wedding songs in the adjacent room of the dark hut, thus drowning the loud sobs of the bride who had been married off "over the mountain and far away", and who from now on would only see her dear ones once a year at the spring festival of Holi, when the daughters return to their home villages. During the handing-over ceremony, the bride not only forfeits her lineage membership, but also her personal or proper name. She will no longer be Gita or be called by the name Gita or be referred to as Gita, unless of course she is fortunate enough to land somewhere outside of family life, perhaps even in proper employment. Otherwise she will be referred to from now on simply by her status, such as by *bahu*, which means daughter-in-law or sister-in-law. Nor are the married couple allowed to call each other by their first names; they refer to each other via a circuitous route, mostly by reference to their children.

When the young married woman has her first menstruation in the *sasuraal* (parents-in-law's house), the Brahman is summoned. The subsequent ceremony is similar to that in which a child receives its name after birth. At the same time this ceremony is the equivalent of the initiation ceremony for boys, for it marks the ritual conclusion of her puberty. (There is a drastic difference here to southern India, where young women celebrate their genuinely first menstruation at their parental home.) The Brahman places a coconut on the young woman's lap after she has remained in isolation for eleven days and taken a purificatory bath every second day. The Brahman sings texts and blesses the coconut in the same way he will do with the newly-born children. On the eleventh day the Brahman takes the new wife to her house and hands her over to her destiny: the continuation of the lineage.

She wears bangles which give her an acoustic accompaniment, her parting is painted red — in analogy to her bleeding vulva — to identify her as a fertile woman, and she wears a long plait which indicates her marital status. In former classical India a plait (*ekveni*) indicated a temporal suspension of the marriage, and only a triple plait (*triveni*) denoted the present state of marriage (Hiltbeitel,1981). With all these signs of her marital status, the young woman documents her subjugation to the new regime, that of her spouse. She gives her "self" up by leaving her "self-ness," as symbolised by her own name, such as Gita, at home at her parents' *ghar*. And when the parents visit her at the *sasuraal*, they have to take along their own (often purely symbolic) food because their daughter, now a stranger, no longer has the right to offer them anything. Rather the daughter must now make her husband her God, as can be read in Manu's text, and moreover every day by preparing his food for him in a pure state and taking his left-overs (*miti*) for her own food, just as is done with the gods when their left-overs (*prasad*) are eaten by the devotees.

Thus the married woman has sacrificed all that previously belonged to her in order to bring herself to the safety of an order that guarantees that she and her children will survive. And now she makes visible sacrifices to this order. She does this without questioning it, and she will also teach her daughters to make this sacrifice, just as she will make it quite clear to her sons what sacrifices they are to expect. These sacrifices provide her with space, at least during the fertile, married stage of her life. She will utilise this space for as long as it is available to her. Its availability ends with the death of her husband, when she passes on to the status of a widow.

"Life loses its flavour," the widows told me in Gahar Banauliya, the village in the foothills of the Himalayas which I visited over a period of seven years, "everything grows dull."

"And," my neighbour there, Sita Devi, added bitterly, "I now simply live on the edge of things. My daughter-in-law says what is to be done." "Don't ask me about it, don't ask," she said, "it's hard." I was struck by the fact that many of the widows were unable to endure our conservations without constantly bursting into tears. They preferred to avoid talking about their reality. It helped them to "live in ignorance of their situation". During the conservations they actually *said* what pained them. It was not easy to take. Conversations of this kind, conversations for the sake of an ethnography, are often an imposition.

After her husband's death — every Hindu woman "wishes" (in official parlance) to die before him — she discards all external signs of her productive life phase. Her red parting is shorn off, her glass bangles and their tinkling sound vanish. Her sandals are removed: she belongs to the house, but the house no longer belongs to her. Her body is no longer permitted any "hot" (warming) spices or meat. On the contrary, she is bound to regular fasts on specific days of the week and at specific times of the day.

She is now under the control of her eldest son, on whom she is dependent. She works for his household and must take instructions for work from her daughter-in-law. Anyone who willingly leaps on to her husband's funeral pyre becomes a *sati*, a goddess who, particularly in Rajasthan, is remembered in the form of memorial stones. There is not a village in Rajasthan without its proud collection of remembrances left by pious *satis* on its walls; while on the way to the funeral pyre on which her departed husband lies waiting, the future *sati* leaves the imprint of her red-painted palm on the wall. The impression is preserved, in both stone and memory. It is repeated on steles that are erected on the edge of the village. "Our *satis*," the chief said to the stranger as if he were talking about an insurance policy, "our *satis* and the good life here in the village, they belong together." The good women, the *satis* and the breast goddesses go to make up the visible discourse on women.

Let us trace the hidden discourse which tells of woman's

power. It is not related or brought up in conversation. One must delve into it to find it. It takes place in the interspaces. It takes place on the fringe of everyday life.

A woman's power holds out promises of happiness, so long as she uses it as only she can. One can go the whole year round to the breast goddesses, who also include the *satis*, for minor problems. But one only goes to the tooth goddess, such as the dreaded Kali, when disaster has already assumed epidemic proportions. The good woman who serves her husband the way Sita did, has her correspondence in the breast goddess. The woman who reflects on all her power and does not control it, does not allow herself constantly to be tamed by father/husband/son, is dramatised in the depictions of the tooth goddesses.

We can learn most clearly how the icon of the tooth goddess originates from everyday affairs from the Indian women who are there where the calamity of everyday life — which has been recast in the idiom of spirit possession — is exorcised: at a Muslim place of pilgrimage, the Mira Datar Dargah. Every story of bewitchment commences at a place of death. The contracts are forged at the graveyard between the person who orders the spell and the *jadukar*, his "magic-maker" (Pfleiderer, 1984). The content of such communications is conveyed by means of menstrual blood. "It was found in his food," the healer (*mujawar*) who attends to the patients at the *dargah* says about "that man who is lying over there in chains after losing his mind". Misfortune is evidently linked directly with the woman's body, from which one should protect oneself.

Similar things are reported from other societies, such as among the Baule in Africa: the women protect themselves from their men by exposing their sex, or by simply threatening to do so. This is a powerful fetish, the men are afraid of it and thus concede the women their space (Luig, 1990). In the village of Gahar Banauliya the men protect themselves from the contamination entailed by childbirth or menstruation by having the women scatter stinging nettles around the bed of the lying-in woman, or live for three days of the month in the cattle shed. In a small ayurvedic clinic near Delhi which housed *unmada* patients (those who have succumbed to madness), Shastriji, the healer, told me that when women are unable to control the heat (*tapas*) in their bodies, or fail to restrain themselves so that the heat in their bodies gains the upper hand, the body does what it wants with them and they end up saying crazy things (Pfleiderer, 1983a).

What the women of Gahar Banauliya have staged in a very convincing manner is the controlled maintenance of an order for which they are responsible and which they pass on. Any deviation from the path of this order is answered with a threat. Not from the unknown, no, but from the woman's body. If a woman does not have it under control, as is assumed when she remains childless, the *danriya* or specialist for possession must be fetched and a *jagar* or therapeutic ritual exorcism has to be employed. The shaman or *danriya* is accompanied by the *jagriya*, the person who knows and sings the texts for order. The de-personalisation of the disorderly woman is staged by these two men in a four-act drama. This is followed by the reconstruction of the woman who lies, rid of the evil, before the ashes of the fire. "So who's the father of the child that the barren woman will now bear?" the visitor from Mumbai asks heretically. And once the men have concluded the ritual they have been instructed to perform and *Golu* the mountain god has departed from the bodies of the possession specialists, the women of the house tug the woman who is buried beneath her sari away from the fire, back into the kitchen. The play, which is called *jagar* (vigil), is over. But the game of the rules continues (Pfleiderer, 1983b). Who instigated this, I ask myself, who is at the back of a thing like this?

As I went to *surya gaun* (sun village), a neighbouring village on the slopes high above, in order to investigate why the women there never grow to be older than 45, I met Gita, Sita Devi's daughter-in-law. I could already see her bright sari shining out to me from the distance, through the Scots pines on the mountain crest. "I'm going to sun village," she calls to me, "to arrange for a jagar." Her *sas* (mother-in-law) is ill.

Gita's wheat flourishes, she has four sons, a beautiful face, and a husband who runs an insurance agency. She masters all the rules. Whenever she became pregnant — repeatedly over the last few years — she sat on the fringe while everyone was dancing at the spring festival *Holi*, or underwent a period of fasting. Now she rules in *her space*. And we can remember where it comes from: life lacks any flavour, Gita's mother-in-law confessed to the ethnographer, when she described *her* (life) space (Pfleiderer, 1987).

And what is assigned to the men?

The Hindu ethnophysiology of ayurveda views life as a continual exchange of substances which even involves death. "Death makes good manure; the most fertile earth is full of corpses" (Egnor, 1983). The male body has developed a very special alchemy in this system. On the basis of the relationship that one hundred drops of urine produce one drop of blood and that one hundred drops of blood produce *one* drop of semen, the male substance may certainly be termed a concentrate. This concentrate is sacred. (One should recall in this context all of the multifarious forms of the *Siva lingam* worship: there is scarcely a Hindu who has not at some time poured a small pot of *ghee*, clarified butter, over the penis (alias *lingam*) of a stone representation of Siva.) And the path to this concentrate is long. No wonder then that one must be careful with it. Spilling it too soon, such as in youth, can easily lead to *gupta roga* (the secret illness of boys in puberty, the nocturnal emission). That this is so is revealed by the numerous discreet signs that can be seen advertising doctors who can alleviate this malady. The order surrounding this very special stuff signifies that is it there for procreation, for the production of sons for the lineage. After concluding this phase of life, the man no longer wastes it on the woman. The male body is so constructed — according to local beliefs — that he may employ the semen in a somewhat better way: it is pumped up into the head "in yogi fashion", as Margaret Egnor writes, (Egnor, 1983) where it is transformed into intelligence or acts to expand consciousness.

The body liquids with which the male body performs the

life-sustaining exchange are mother's milk and its own semen. It receives such an abundance of the former that it is hard to imagine that it will manage to get away without a severe dependency syndrome after it is weaned. And as we know, the traditional regulations governing marriage have arranged things in such a way that the man will never leave his mother. That is the way in the Hindu joint-family model. And his semen produces for him his son, to whom he will also be bound in the next twist of the Hindu karmic voyage. He only sets out on it if the son, who accompanies him to the beyond and lights his funeral pyre, is from his own seed.

If that's the case, I think to myself, the man must be utterly at the mercy of a chaste woman. Not only can she physically ruin a man (think of the poor fellow who lost his reason after a woman mixed menstrual blood in his food), no, she can also give him the false code, in karmic terms, and damn him to roam aimlessly for all eternity. For that is what would happen if his son were not really *his* son. Women understand man's dependency on them, as is clearly shown by the dictates of the body fluids. When women *speak* of their boundaries, those that are set down by society, they simultaneously *think* of their power, which lies at the bottom of it all. The key word here is *prakrti*. Some of the orthodox directions in Hindu philosophy bear eloquent witness to this. The ayurvedic cosmology has, for instance, echoes of *Samkhya* philosophy. This is described concisely by Margaret Egnor (1983):

> "... the cosmos and each person are formed of two components: a female component, or *Prakrti*, which forms the body, and a male component or *Purusa*, which is the soul. *Purusa* is indivisible, atomic and immutable, but *Prakrti* has parts and is subject to change.
>
> The cosmos comes into existence when *Purusa* impregnates *Prakrti* with his essence. Then *Prakrti*, who previously had been in a state of internal balance, is thrown into disequilibrium, and proceeds to evolve the universe (and the body) from varying combinations of the different components (the three *gunas*) of herself. *Purusa*, being unchanging, is also non-productive. *Prakrti* creates out of her own substance; her ability to change (become other) is her ability to create. *Purusa* does not participate in the

> evolution of the body/cosmos, but only observes it, as a prisoner within it.
>
> Although *Purusa* is conscious and *Prakrti* not, the Ayurvedic texts tell us that *Purusa*, being a non-participant in the life process, is indifferent to pleasure and pain, whereas *Prakrti* is not. *Purusa* only thinks he feels pleasure and pain inasmuch as he is bound to *Prakrti* and identifies himself with her. According to the text *Samkhya-karika*, when the creation is completed and *Purusa* has watched *Prakrti* evolve the body around him, he sees himself in her mirror and realizes he is different from her. Then *Prakrti*, having fulfilled her function, returns to her original undifferentiated, unmanifest state, and *Purusa* is free again."

Ayurvedic physiology continues this story of the act of creation. It says that the female body can produce descendants without outside assistance. It merely requires the male substance in order to bring about the differentiation. (This could also be interpreted as genetic material.) The male element in the newly forming body is the permanent framework, such as the hair, bones and nails. The lighter parts of the foetus come from the mother. Consequently the constitution of a body is also termed *prakrti*, which is formed in turn from the three *dosas* (*vata, pitta* and *kapha*, wind, bile and mucus). *Dosa* means error, being ill, or suffering. Its basic characteristic is change, as is also the case with prakrti. The ayurvedic model of life and death designates the male part as an immutable (and intransformable) soul and the female part as a constantly changing body which houses the male part. Change brings about life — and death, which liberates the soul.

This excursion into worlds physiological should not be concluded without taking a look at the most alchemical of all theses. The physiological equivalent of the liberation of the soul can be seen in the impetus of the cleansing process among the body elements. And here the male seed, as already noted, has the longest way to go. It is also distinguished from the other bodily substances by yet another dimension: it is indivisible and "like gold purified a thousand times".

So, just as menstrual blood teaches man the meaning of fear, his seed is highly coveted: by himself for expanding his techniques of consciousness in "yogi fashion", and by the woman in order to create the much desired son. Hindu psychology has a parable at the ready for this, which has been reframed by the psychoanalyst Sudhir Kakar. This says that the bounteous attention bestowed by the mother on the male baby (triggered by a lack of self-esteem because woman belongs to the less desirable or female sex), and which does not even stop at erotic expressions of this fondness, leaves such a lasting impression on the boy that he retreats, intimidated, from the sexually mature woman and turns to younger women (Kakar,1978). He views the older, more mature woman within the framework of the tooth goddesses. She nourished him with milk. And now he must keep her alive with his semen; he must "feed" her in order to prevent her from flying into a rage.

This inversion of the Hindu model of life brings these descriptions of the relation between the sexes, as based on the transformation of vital fluids and functions, full circle.

Women are not controlled by men, as I already maintained at the beginning, rather women control women by maintaining the petrifying Hindu family model in order to create — at a sacrifice — a safe life space for themselves. The rigidity of this model is undermined by the ayurvedic theory of the body. This points to the genuine, female vitality which is often grasped simply as a ruse of helplessness. This dysfunctionality of a social institution can be evaluated by the way it overevaluates its inversions.

And yet the woman gives the man what belongs to man, if only via fasting and a representative gaze in the reversed direction. Let us look at the following ritual, one that is performed regularly. The scene quite literally deludes the man into believing that he is and remains the *divine* spouse.

"It reminds us of our wedding," says Parvati, who lives in a small town in Rajasthan. "But we perform it every month. *Paramparah*," she says, by which she means tradition. When everyone, children, husband, mother-in-law and brother-in-law, has left the kitchen, fully fed and satisfied, she enters the courtyard with her clay jug. "I haven't eaten a thing all day, you know, because today's *purnima ka vrat* (the full-moon fast) which I always observe. We fast the whole day long. Until the full moon starts to show itself. Once that point has arrived, we fill the clay jug brimful with water and observe the rising moon over the brim. We are not allowed to look at the moon directly. And then the mirror image of the moon, *chandra ma*, appears on the water in my jug. I walk round it seven times, just as at my wedding. And then I break my fast," she says. "I do it in order to keep my *pati dev* (divine spouse) alive and in good health."

She does not look at the moon directly, but encircles it while it is reflected in the water jug. The jug is the symbol of the uterus, of life. When a Hindu is cremated, a clay jug is smashed by his head — before his body is consumed by the flames — to symbolise the end of his life. When Turkish women are barren they continue to bury empty clay pots until they conceive. The moon is the image for the female fertility cycle. The moon also stands for the night, the dark side, the spiritual and the "unofficial" side of things. The symbolism of the ritual which Parvati showed me solely recalls woman, her spirituality and her fertility. But what Parvati *said* to me in her words spoke solely of her husband, of his well-being, his fertility. This double talk, the unofficial side *within* the ritual and the official side *about* the ritual, this double discourse, is precisely what we wish to track down here.

The women whom I encountered live fully in the knowledge that the pressure imposed on them by the dysfunctional Hindu family model can be unbearable or even deadly. In this chapter I have described a few coordinates which determine the spaces traditionally accorded to women. In the following chapters we shall sound out those spaces to which women escape when they are no longer able to stand up to the everyday rules.

Chapter 3

The Question, the Journey and the Field

In this chapter I shall describe the way I personally approached the question about the actual state of possession and the medium of trance, which is to say the state which women use as their unofficial space and which nevertheless remains a part of everyday life in India. The conversations and the travels which helped me during my discoveries will crop up in this chapter, as will some of the people I talked with. As I have already hinted, my concern in this book is the *everyday nature* of altered states of consciousness, its social status, and its common usage during crises. In this chapter I will give some insight into the life of the anthropologist performing his or her fieldwork, and into the experiences which I share with so many of my colleagues, both male and female, but which few ever describe. A notable exception is, among one or two others, Michael Moffat's book on several groups of untouchables in southern India, in which he writes openly in the introduction about his own state of mind ("I had fits of insanity") while attempting to live a day-to-day existence with the group he wished to write about (Moffat, 1979). I shall write on my marvellous interpreter, whom I shall name Vikram Nath in my text, and without whom I would never have been able to conduct these conversations during the years in which I was still speechless and neither spoke nor understood Hindi. Later, once I had become linguistically autonomous, he continued his unflagging work with me as we collected the data on the Mira Datar Dargah.

But let us look at the journey which took me to the Mira Datar Dargah and opened up many questions to me about women in India in particular, and women in a patriarchy in general.

The Question

Let us begin with a university lecture:

Silence. "That concludes my lecture," says the foreign speaker, an Indian. The audience looks at him attentively. An audience of Indologists and anthropologists, the majority are students, a few are their lecturers, including myself. Who will ask the first question, and what will they ask?

The topic is possession. I have jotted down my interest in this subject in my diary. This helps jog my memory. The portly Dr. Rocquefort, who always starts to vibrate whenever Indian music is played, asks whether the lecturer had always been able to tell who caused the possession and whether it was genuine. The person doing the asking does not "know" what "it" is, I continue jotting, he hasn't a clue, he'd do better to stay away from lectures like this. "The mountain spirit, he's called Golu, he causes the possession," the lecturer replies simply. He looks slightly disappointed.

But before the lecturer succumbs to further disappointments over such questions, Gilbert, one of our most popular lecturers whom everyone can call by his first name, and who had also invited the Indian speaker in the first place, says: "Even cults of possession are commonplace in India. Nobody is surprised when someone goes into a trance beside them. For Hindus it is part of their devotion to a personal god to fall into an ecstasy like that. People fight and argue with their god. And they also fall into a trance for him and through him," he says. Gilbert is well-liked among the students. We enjoy the way he acknowledges the normality of things which our culture has long since felt the need to exclude. We like his findings because he has integrated his experiences in India into his normal life.

Am I still interested in possession, someone asks me, handing me a newspaper report across the table of a young woman in Franconia who was tortured and starved to death by her priest, who thought she was possessed by the devil. The case of Anneliese Michel, I read, has yet to be closed; exhumation, question mark. It happened near Würzburg. The last "witch" was burned at Bamberg, not long ago, I think, and am surprised at the Franconians, whom I grew up quite close to. No, I answer, I am looking for something else, something that goes further, something that's alive.

I continue to follow my thread. I want to know what possession is. But I want to know it in a way that is "different" to the meta-level of description. I want to know what the discourse on possession is like there, where it is practised. Obviously in India, obviously in Africa, as a simply endless pile of literature has meanwhile come to suggest. And I want to know just how this discourse provokes a complementary ongoing discourse which acts to exclude the subject and banish it to marginal spaces. Later, in the eighties, marvellous studies were to appear on possession and possession specialists, but these were not yet available to us in the seventies. I discovered that my questions were echoed in Gananath Obeyesekere's *Medusa's Hair* and in *Boiling Energy* by Richard Katz, as well as in Bruce Kapferer's *A Celebration of Demons* and the film on the Balinese medium Jero Tapakan by Timothy Asch and Linda O'Connor.

The first of these reports is on the day-to-day life of religious virtuosi (in Weber's sense), their existential crises and their way back into a new life as spiritual experts and healers. The location is present-day Sri Lanka. The ethnographer is one of the most conscientious and resourceful I know. The second book reports on the !Kung San of the Kalahari Desert in southern Africa, and how their life energy, *num*,[1] rises and puts them into a trance; the energy catapults them across the cosmos and, if they do not stop and cool down in good time and leave the circle of the singers and people in trance, they may even experience death.

Both of these books reveal this journey out of oneself, outside of one's self, as part of the human condition, as something intrinsically and universally human.

The third work, a detailed ethnographic study of possession which also focuses on Sri Lanka, describes the inner and outer, i.e. the mental and social geography of the occurrence. Kapferer examines the social crisis — which, through the fact of possession, becomes a psycho-social drama — from the position of each of the protagonists. He allows everyone involved to have their say, and with that is able to portray the destructive side of demonic possession as an inversion of the prevailing culture, and to trace the routes along which the evil is healed in the form of rituals.

A fourth work, the film and the accompanying book by the ethnographer Linda O'Connor and the film-maker Timothy Asch, centres on the work of the medium Jero Tapakan (Asch, O'Connor et al, 1986). The word *work* is meant here in the sense of real craftsmanship. And the Balinese healer Jero Tapakan views her work as just that, as she conveys to the audience during the film when she discusses her work with the ethnographer while watching the film material. For some her astonishment at her appearance during the trance she enters in order to earn her money is "proof", for others a successful link-up between the discourses on trance and within trance, i.e. text and metatext. Let us take a look at this film:

Jero Tapakan summons her helping spirits with a metallic voice. She invites them to enter her body, and asks for their assistance. She loses herself while doing so, but remains there as a vessel. The authors describe her as a spirit medium, the village inhabitants as a balian. She is regarded as a dependable *balian.* In her culture in Bali trance is part of everyday life, as it is in India and Africa. People work with it, in it. It happens. It comes about. It is summoned. And that is what the outside observer discovers while watching. Since I, too, have seen and experienced this, I would like to give my own report on it, taken from my travel diary during my field research in the mountain village in Uttar Pradesh:

Golu, Goril or Goraknath is a mountain spirit. He inhabits the mountain range before the main crest of the Himalayas. Much has been written about him in the anthropological writings of Indians, Britons and others. I got to know him while living in the Nainital district with the object of reporting on the lives of the farming women. The women paid no attention to him. They preferred Siva and Hanuman and fasted for each of them once a week, on Tuesdays and Mondays respectively. But their *danriya*, their possession specialist whom I came across there during my first visit, an old vagabond from the Brahman caste by the name of Kanial, numbered him among his work gods when with his assistance he went into a trance in order to conduct a therapeutic session for the village inhabitants. They call that *jagar khelna*. During this the spectators said: "Look, it's Sem now, and now it's Golu, yes, Golu has come to him." And as proof that Golu had entered him, Kanial leapt into the glowing ashes with a loud cry and placed his head on the edge of the fire that had been lit for the *jagar*. "I cannot see Golu," I wrote in my diary: "The noise of the ritual gets in the way." A few days later I went with Jagdish, the husband of a neighbour, to the temple festival of Golu. Jagdish wants to sacrifice a goat. He grins as he says, "She will walk all the way there in front of me, and come back lying on my shoulders." An abbreviation of the principle of sacrifice. We start up the steep grassy hills before daybreak. It's some twenty kilometres away, even though the small, white temple complex is visible from our valley. Scot's pines line the crests of the hill and shield us from the rising sun. As we make our way up we can see other people on the hills around, bringing their sacrifices to the temple: coconuts, rice, fruit, plants and above all goats. Lots of goats. They emit lengthy bleats. Some are carried by all fours, and their bleats turns into cries, screams. Once inside the temple courtyard we see on the far side of the grass-covered ground, which is traversed by stone paths, a large gathering which has come with goats. This is the place of slaughter. The *pujari* severs the goats' necks with a single blow. Blood spurts and flows out of the temple along small runnels and then on down the path on the side of the hill. Or so I had imagined the sacrificial victims' ascent to the pyramids, forced to walk towards the downward flow of blood, when as a schoolgirl I read the book by the blind author Prescott on the conquest of Tenochtitlan (Mexico). The uneasiness of the flocks of goats that were being driven towards the place of slaughter was quite understandable. Jagdish placed his goat on his shoulders and carried it over to the small Golu shrine. Niam, Jagdish's wife, told me the evening before while kneading and frying chapattis for our picnic: "You only have to leave its thighs there. Tomorrow evening we'll have goat stew."

My legs felt hollow and empty at the thought of this, everything turned grey before my eyes and I felt waves of nausea rising up inside me because I had not eaten breakfast and my stomach felt queasy. But then Golu appeared and the veil vanished from my eyes. He had selected one of the pilgrims from town for his manifestation.

We had already seen the small, delicate man with his grey stubbly hair as he climbed the mountain in front of us with his goat and his bundle of offerings and food for the journey. He had stood in line with us. Was in front of us. He knelt before the small window through which Golu's image, a small stone figure painted in dark colours and blackened by the soot of the oil lamps, could be seen. He placed his portion of goat meat before the window niche. And handed a small sack of rice into the window which was received by the hands of the *pujari*. He raised his folded hands and immersed himself in prayer. At first he murmured old, time-honoured sentences. But then a sound of singing rose from his mouth and in that same moment his whole body began to tremble fiercely. His body bobbed up and down until his upper body started to perform a succession of elastic bounds in a squatting position. The motion was so fast that all that could be seen of him was a haze. He raised his hands while simultaneously looking as though he was about to succumb once and for all to this trembling. And then it subsided, this thing that had overcome him. "He is possessed by God, by Golu," a man from the plains suddenly bellowed into my ear, a man who spoke English and felt the need to explain things to me. What a shame that I was white. What a shame that this caused me to be given this explanation.

The man emerged from his transformation and looked about him in astonishment, as if awakening, and then looked the idol in the eyes and muttered a formula that no one could hear. His eyes still revealed the ecstasy he must have experienced while the presence of the god Golu had set his body into such rhythms and into a trance so deep that it had cut him off totally from his surroundings for three or four whole minutes, allowing him to sink completely into his mystic experience. The eyes of the god must have overcome him. Overcome, then possessed, and then in trance, that was the sequence. Trance, which comes from *transire* (Latin to go across), is what one sees when a supernatural being comes and occupies a human body.

Van Gennep, an author who is presented to every young student of anthropology as the great scholar who described the psychological and sociological stages of ritual, foresaw such sequences. But much more occurred here. What happened as the man's body escaped its owner and became simply a heaving mass? Had it left the temporal and spatial coordinates of our cultural experience? Had his mind, his soul, broken through the limitations created by the category of thought? Had he experienced for a fraction of a second the stream of timelessness flowing through the universe? Had he transcended the apparent boundaries that determine the individual, so as to break out into a metaphysical reality and become one with the basis of the entirety of existence, or with the Beyond that signifies the unity of all life? And while I am arranging all this into words, I realise that this will end up with the man's experience being locked away from us. That is the customary way of dealing with such phenomena in the academic world. And that must have been extremely difficult for the lecturer in the seminar room mentioned earlier: the necessity of locking up what has been experienced, what had been seen and was allegedly so alien, into words, when faced with those "how and why" questions.

The academic world, which has difficulties leaving the universe of Newton and Descartes, has assembled a canon of words that has to fit to everything that is experienced and perceived emotionally. Even the mathematical formulae that represent the physicist's experiences during his experiments are merely one-dimensional portraits of the events that actually took place before the scientist's eyes. Added to which, the representation is culturally specific, like every set of findings in science (Latour and Wolgar, 1979). Obviously anthropology, the science of culture, has no additional spaces to offer than other sciences, nor has it woven a broader mesh into its perceptual net. For in every discipline people simply make the knowledge that they require — into knowledge. He who pays the piper calls the tune: whose knowledge?

I once went to a conference of social scientists and South Asia experts. I wanted to know who was looking into the day-to-day experience of trance in India. I wanted to get to know people who had tackled this.

Everything that the people from the West noticed about the differences that could be seen out there in India was presented at this conference in the form of workshops and papers. And it kept being presented at lots of other conferences of the same kind. And what was presented? The disconcerting aspects of the Other. For India that was always the caste system, in all its permanence and fragility. The ruling discourse's assumptions about the Other are tucked away behind titles like "Continuity and Change". Just as the earth-shattering news about of the Hindu woman's life-stages is spread by women from the scientific community in their scientific talk about the women there. And in the same way, the ascent of the untouchables after their exodus from their villages kept being brought up. After opting out of the relationship prescribed by the caste system came the relationship prescribed by the new economy, which leads to the industrial estates of the big cities. Continuity and change? Everyone remains unchanged, true to his or her reality.

One ought to be able to reverse the ethnographic eye, at least that was my wish at this conference. The people who we keep turning, quite matter-of-factly, into ethnographic objects must come and visit us and reverse the process. It would have to be someone who is free of our mental restraints and can investigate *our* culture from the standpoint of his Indian notions.

I found this man after five years and numerous journeys to India. His name was Ramnath Kumar and he came from Bihar. He had the sharpest of ethnographic eyes and knew how to read our culture.

Later, after we had finished our work in India, I invited this Indian friend — who had to put up with the title of research assistant during our work — to Germany. Once he was back home with his wife, who had been found for him by his parents, he wrote a book about Germany. He wrote about the children who are left on their own by their parents, at precisely the point when they begin to grow up. About the parents' dogs, which remind them that the house had once been full of children and noise. He wrote about people seated on a park bench; three days had passed and still they had not found anyone who would talk with them. And he calculated that the insurance on my oil tank cost as much in one year as the financial support he sent his aged parents in his village. He wrote away the chill that beset his body in Germany. There are no conferences in *his country* on the topics that astonished *him*. There are four thousand years of Brahmanism behind the self-evident way he found his bearings, a Brahmanism in which he first found himself again as he began writing the book, which also came to be published and read.

The cafeteria acts as the bazaar at this conference. Indian visitors have focussed their conversations on our astonishment. Indian anthropologists have become masters in the way in which *we* ask questions. They have adopted our process of scientific inquiry with perfection and employ its instruments with such precision that they now play an equal part in this game of estrangement and distortion. The exceptions to this are few and far between: representative here is the outstanding ethnographer and anthropologist Gananath Obeyesekere.[2] His work on the concept of depression and the Buddhist image of man countered a fashion in research that had assumed absurd dimensions, and at a point when the level of agreement was starting to get dangerous. His work gave a timely corrective to the American "be-happy" psychology.

Sitting in the cafeteria was Dr.Shah, a renowned sociologist from north India. Our meeting was occasioned by a chance introduction. "You want to study trance and possession in India?" he asked me, making quite sure that he had understood me correctly. And his very query had so little to do with my initial question that I didn't ask the man again. Particularly because his answer harboured a threat: "That's hard to find nowadays in India, and if you really want to do that it will take a lifetime." That is the best threat that a Hindu can make to a European, the threat of the dwindling time in this one single life. Dr. Shah knew trance. There is no one in India who does not know or see it. But he had made his experiences invisible to himself and placed them at a safe distance when he said, "on top of which there is a lot of superstition...".

The conference was lovely because it was held by the sea and offered lots of beer parties, but I didn't get any further with my question.

The question about everyday experiences in and of trance, which can be seen in the literature of the eighties, occupied a lot of people's attention at that time. But only ten years later were the conferences to provide the cross-connections that would have helped them. Consequently, Maya Deren's peerless document *Divine Horsemen* on Haitian trance, written in the fifties, remained our sole model. The body in trance is ridden by an *ioa*, a ghost. The person's gaze is directed inwards in a way that likewise overcomes anyone who looks at this person who is so overcome. The gaze of the Golu worshipper who sacrificed his goat was likewise inwardly directed while his body bobbed and bounced up and down.

When it came to my own, personal interest in trance in day-to-day India, my invisible helping hand turned out to be Hiranand, who was sitting there in my office, which handles the scholarships for the institute, as I returned. He knew all about trance, had studied it while becoming an anthropologist in Vienna, and it was there that he discovered that what he knew was of interest. Of academic interest. He admitted to this interest by refusing to let the Other, his experience back home with the bopas,[3] be stamped as superstition and assigned it to the fringes of his experience. Rather, he held on to it as hard information that would be of help. This not only made him unusual, but also a valuable source for both himself and others. Once the work we shared in the office had come to an end and he had found a job for himself and his wife in India, I went and visited him before his return. "What you're looking for is to be found on every street corner there. You simply have to take a walk. Take a walk, and best of all with Vikram Nath." What he meant was take a walk around the villages of Gujarat. From one small shrine on the wayside to the next. That is what he meant. And after he had flown to India and I to North Africa to complete a project, I received a postcard from him with a picture of Ganesh[4] on the other side. Ganesh is good at the beginning. And dependable.

The Journey

India was never one of my subjects while I was a student; the things that I associated with it prevented me from making any contact with it. As I recalled from the books and tales of my childhood, things there were governed by higher powers. And the Indian way of life, such as one surmised and indeed heard, or sensed and saw on meeting Indians at parties, conferences, in trains or on planes, was not designed to make one ask any further.

I became acquainted with India through the Hindi movie. I read in the newspaper that Indian film-goers skipped their main meals noticeably often in order to go to a film. As a child I wanted nothing more than to go to the one cinema in our small town, and would have sacrificed any number of meals to do so. These Indians interested me. Cinema, a national passion? I wanted to see that. That was my real interest in the country. What films did they make and watch? What were the melodies they sung on the streets, what were they looking for in the cinema? Or, I wondered, what were they fleeing from? What did the film do to them, what did they do with the film?

I applied for research funding so that I could see all the films in India that evidently engrossed the people there. I learned the language of the film before I got to know that of the people, although in the final analysis it was also the language of the people. First of all I took in the films that the homesick Pakistanis watched on Sunday mornings in German cinemas. Poverty, fraternal hatred and motherly love, reconciliation and illness, blood and death. Happiness and disaster. String music that cut the listener to the quick and carried the over-exaggerated metaphors of everyday India through the plot, until the final denouement of the interminable drama allowed the tortured spectator to exit from the belly of the cinema. Torture instead of trance? The application for a study into "Audience Reactions to Hindi Films" was accepted. I flew to India in order to go to the cinema and live and experience daily life in front of the silver screen. Because, if Dr. Shah was right and it is quite impossible to come across (spirit) possession, at least I would meet up with people who were *ob*sessed with the cinema.

I began visiting the cinema with an Indian family and by sharing their obsession with films. Afterwards they spoke to me on my tape recorder. And after the German Embassy allowed me to use their cinemobile, the project became even more efficient. We could now drive from village to village with one of the Hindi movie hits, *Do Raaste* or "Two Paths", project it to the villagers and discuss the content. The content is enthralling. It describes an Indian family which is split in two. The one half, the "good half" in the film, remains faithful to the traditions, shuns modernity and consequently becomes impoverished. The other half is led by the daughter-in-law, who has abandoned the traditions and gained a degree abroad. The spectator is whipped up against her because she is depicted as a tooth goddess, while the good daughter-in-law corresponds to the Sita ideal. The village inhabitants in Uttar Pradesh thought that the film was worth seeing — many had never even seen one before. But they told us that it would be more profitable for us foreigners to visit one of their own weddings and get to know India as it really is. We wrote a book about it all which was published in Delhi in 1985 by Manohar Book Service under the title: *The Hindi Film: agent and reagent of cultural change?* It was widely read and sold well because our European inquisitiveness constituted a highly entertaining and exotic ethnographicum for the Indians.[5] Perhaps its success was also due to the fact that it became the mirror of what the strangers' gaze was able to explain. The book's message was simple but convincing. A visit to the cinema assumes the place of a pilgrimage in both the ritual and day-to-day manner in which it is performed. And the similarity between a pilgrimage and a visit to the cinema was not merely superficial, for it was also functional. The actors look the spectator direct in the eye. They reach him by becoming his alter. An oversized, over-exaggerated, often over-powerful and over-powering alter. The eye contact, even if it is just assumed, transfers to the spectator what he believes to be in it. Power, superiority, goodness: the string of fantasies is never-ending. But although wickedness is also presented face on, is so clearly underlined and partitioned that one would never take to it, not even by accident.

"Ravana, the representative of evil in the *Ramayana*, is always black in both his clothes and his soul, and this errant son always flourishes an outsized whisky bottle in his hand, if not two," wrote my co-author Lothar Lutze after we had once again spent half a day working in a *bombaihindiphilum*.[6] It is this eye-to-eye situation that gives the Hindi film its success across all the state borders and every caste barrier. It is immediately comprehensible and plausible. It is a repetition and through this repetition a secularisation of the way a person in prayer beholds a picture of God.

In Mumbai I turned to Vikram Nath on Hiranand's recommendation, for I only knew the districts of the thieves, rogues and millionaires from films. He came to the airport. His glasses concealed a pair of clever eyes. His broad grin revealed his addiction. Betel. His mouth kept a dark red liquid in constant motion, just allowing fleeting glances of his white teeth. The likes of that have yet to be shown in a Hollywood Dracula film. The sight was so inscrutable that it forestalled any questions. Vikram Nath took me to his wife and family for supper. I wouldn't have expected either the one or the other when I first set eyes on him. But he had both. And that's why he had to offer his services, even though he found the thought of daily work quite unbearable. He had settled on a job description that left everything open and opened many possibilities: "anthropologist's field guide". I knew "field guides" from the literature, in the sense of manuals. These describe the procedures for asking questions and for waiting for the right moment, as well as what to do in the gaps between those moments, when gathering anthropological data — which curiously is called field work, even though it is mostly performed in rooms. Vikram Nath was an *active* field guide who from one moment to the next gave the right prompts to the anthropologist. Before me he had guided a number of German-speaking anthropology professors through "interesting regions" and been astonished, as he told me, at their questions.

Hiranand had already clued him in on me. "She wants to know all there is to know about trance and possession from Mumbai to Ahmedabad," he had told him. "It would best if you went by foot." We were having breakfast in the YMCA in Mumbai. Vikram Nath presented me with a programme which might just be the right thing, he said, to whet my curiosity. Then he described the latest films from postmodern German filmmakers like Rainer Werner Fassbinder and asked me to fill in the missing contexts for him. His face dropped as I told him about my Sunday morning experiences in the latest Hindi films. That was not what he wanted to hear. "My children sing all the latest hits from the films," he said in a friendly but resigned way as he realised that I was no expert on the German film. He's not interested in what interests me, I noted in turn, so I proceeded to our mutual task.

The next day we went off to look at a sample, it seemed, of what he was offering: a shrine that attracts those who "labour and are heavy laden". We get on a bus which reminds me for a few minutes of London, for we sit upstairs. But not for long because then we change buses and travel for over half an hour through inhabited pavements, Indian villages on municipal tarmac, slums built along the road like a never-ending campsite. The women have hung up their saris between the tents to dry. And other items of laundry, lots of small pieces of laundry, can be seen hanging from the children who have grown up among these rows of tents.

After travelling for an hour we get out at a market for secondhand metal goods. The street is ruled by human freight carriers. Two-wheeled carts filled with iron parts are tugged through the traffic by one or two men who literally shout their way through the incredible commotion: "Get out of the way, now," they shout, but often in vain, so the alternative is to steer the load with all its weight directly at the obstacle, which often has better results. As pedestrians we are forced to stick to a labyrinthine route which Vikram Nath seems to have planned and paced out in advance. We ask the way to a place called *Mira Sayed Ali Datar Dargah Sharif,*[7] and are directed to a muddy alley full of puddles and bordered by wooden huts. Some of them have been turned into shops or tea-stalls. Standing about the alley are fruit traders with hand carts. A bunch of bananas costs four rupees when Vikram Nath does the buying, but eight if I do. But this world order is justifiable because the white men simply have more of what the banana-sellers lack. And since it is rupees that highlight this difference, I have no alternative but to go along with this form of redistribution.

Our attention is drawn to a building with a corrugated iron roof at the end of the alley by a green pennant fluttering above the entrance on a pole. Green, the colour of Islam, time and again, often on the roadside and indicating the presence of a tiny tomb, and more importantly showing that this is Muslim territory. We deposit our shoes with one of the custodians at the entrance for a few paise and are received by *mujawars,*[8] the dignitaries of the place. Only Vikram Nath is allowed to visit the tomb inside, for women have to remain in the surrounding hall. If the grave is of a woman, the opposite is true, as we were later to discover. The grave itself is decked with flowers, mostly roses or rose petals scattered over red and green velvet. It seems that a lot of people come here. We are told that it will be full in the afternoon, and return several hours later, following the visitors who trail along the small muddy alley to the shrine. This time the halls around the tomb are full of people. The air is heavy with incense, piercing screams echo through the rooms. Several women are throwing themselves energetically on to their hands so that their palms slap against the floor while their loose hair flies through the air. Others are standing nearby, unconcerned by this, their faces turned to the grave while muttering verses from the Koran. The dignitaries touch the visitors or *sawwalis*[9] with a bunch of peacock feathers and hand them a glass of holy water to drink. After a while the people who were sunk in prayer return to themselves and make their way to the exit. The women who have entered a state of inner dissolution slump down and remain crouching for a while in a curled-up position, concealed under their saris or *dupattas*.[10] Then they gather their belongings and their wits, get up and leave, almost sauntering, for the exit. We also leave.

"What's that?" I ask Vikram Nath in the bus. "That is just the local branch," he replies, "the actual temple is north of Gujarat, at least a day's journey from here. According to legend, Mira Sayed Ali was a Muslim martyr five hundred years ago. His grave is in Gujarat. The devout often go there and bring back consecrated stones in order to build a small replica of the tomb as a place of daily pilgrimage. These local shrines are called *chillas*.[11] We were in one just now." "So the grave is not a real grave then?" I ask in astonishment. "The grave," he replies impatiently, "is in Gujarat, just as I said." "And this one here?" I ask. "Is not a grave," he answers curtly. We agree in the end that it stands for the real grave, and are satisfied that we have established this sign for us.

Did I want to see something like that, he asked me searchingly. "Yes, that would be just the thing," I reply. I am still confronted with what for me is a contradiction: the way the women had rolled about on the floor moaning, pleading, and emitting blood-curdling screams, and then suddenly got up, utterly transformed, found their bearings once again in the world and left the sanctuary merrily with their shopping in their hand. "How is that possible?" I ask myself. I direct my question to Vikram Nath: "It's always like that, it's nothing special. The women simply have a *hajri*.[12] That means presence.

The same word is used at school when the teachers checks whether everyone is present. *Hajri*, the teacher says, please *hajri*, please say if you're there, and the pupils obey. Here in the shrine a *bhut* or *balla* is present in the women. That is what the word *hajri* refers to. *Hajri ati*, with me it ends in *hajri*, the women say when they want people to know that they are dealing with a spirit, and a fairly evil one at that, that is inside them. "And why only women, why doesn't one see men like that?" I continue with my questions. "Men have it as well, but they do not say so or they say instead that they have a silent presence, a *ghum hajri*."[13] "So they don't have to scream anything out of their system," I think out loud, but I receive no answer.

It is the women mourners who feel the need to scream everything out of their system, and even back home in our small town it was always the women at the burials who were allowed to wail, rather than the men.

"This is something that I would really like to look into," I say to Vikram Nath, who then sets about making suggestions for our journey.

We take the night train to the north, to the town of Balsar in the southern-most district of the state of Gujarat. This is my first train journey in India, and Vikram Nath must have felt more like a nurse-maid than interpreter, what with all of my questions which circled exclusively around the realms of nutrition, bodies and hygiene. As the train sets off my first impressions are dominated by the swarms of traders, salesmen and shoe-shines who invade the carriage while the passengers make their way to their seats or, in our case, our sleeping berths, with mostly as much effort as luggage. No sooner has my interest been caught by the siren call of a banana seller (*kela-kele-ek rupea teeeeein*, bananas, bananas, three for a rupee) than he is replaced by a tea boy who balances a tank of tea and a bucket full of glasses on his head and works his way through the passengers who have settled in. Scarcely able to account for my actions amid all this variety, I must have nodded in response to the shoe-shine's question "shoe shine sir", for as I look down I discover that he had already spread out his tools before my feet. After finishing his work, he takes his money and hides it in a shoe cream tin for safe-keeping.

The next morning we arrive at Balsar and go to the bus stop. While queuing for the bus — the boarding points are ringed in by iron rails to keep the queue in line — a large crowd of young men, as well as several boys and a few women, gathers around us and stares silently and insistently at me. A dead dog is lying there before the bus. It is dragged away on a string that someone ties to its hind paw. The rush makes boarding almost impossible. We drive to a village called Talao Chora. We pass a small hut, and from inside comes a song recital that is interrupted by muttering from a number of voices. "That's Bhanabhai," we are told by the people we ask. He receives visitors on Mondays and Thursdays. We are in luck, today is Thursday. We ask if we may enter and sit among the congregation of singers. Later as Vikram Nath and I documented and published our travel experiences, we described Bhanabhai as follows...

The Field

"In Talao Chora near Balsar, Gujarat, an agricultural labourer from the village who calls himself Bhanabhai and regards himself as one of the *Halapati* group, practices every Monday and Thursday from nine a.m. till one p.m. in a temple area that was erected one year ago. After briefly invoking the spirit *Ram Deo Pir* with the aid of incense, the possession specialist Bhanabhai goes into trance. He sits on a cushion, sways his hips, turns his back to his audience and recites a song with a set structure. The Ram Deo Pir movement comes from Rajasthan, where Bhanabhai also learned the songs, the texts, trance and its use for diagnostic purposes from his guru." (Becker-Pfleiderer and Dharamsey, 1978)

We feel that he is a "hybrid" type of healer who uses his empirical knowledge of herbs from ayurvedic medicine just as equally as possession by Ram Deo Pir.

The encounter with Bhanabhai ended up as a "finding" in a work that endeavoured to classify what had been seen and what had occurred, and to categorize this under differing forms of medical and therapeutic traditions (ibid, p.59). But it is impossible to learn what really happened from this kind of publication. It would be useful for a start to know more about the person who was at the back of it when Bhanabhai fell into a trance in his hut and sang his nasal song before his congregation. Because all we know is that Ram Deo Pir, the saint from Rajasthan who at the back of it, is a miracle-worker.

Later on, while travelling to Ramdeovara in Rajasthan in order to pick up the saint's trail, I discovered a man called Makkhanlal at Ram Deo Pir's place of burial, which became a place of worship, who told me:

"Ram Deo Pir was a miracle-worker, and the miracles were such that five sages in Mecca heard of his fame and came to Ramdeovara in order to see what he did with their own eyes. They found a youth who was sitting there, cleaning his teeth with a *neem* twig. Was he Ram Deo Pir, they asked. The young Ram sent them away on a humorous whim with the words 'you'll find him over there', and with that he quickly stuck his *neem* twig in the ground. As the sages returned to him after being unable to find the saint elsewhere, they were astonished at this enormous tree.[14]

Yet they wanted more miracles from him and said, 'We're hungry, terribly hungry, can't you give us something to eat,' to which Ram answered, 'Allow me to invite you to a meal.' And five trees grew before their eyes, all covered with food. But because the sages required more miracles before they would acknowledge him as a saint, they said: 'And if there were more of us, six people or twelve or twenty-four, could you still feed us?' And twenty-four trees covered in food grew up out the ground as if by a miracle," said Makkhanlal, as well as others who in the meantime had come and sat down with us. Makkhanlal formulated his personal god by jotting down the following equation in his notebook:

Ram — Avatar God Ram
Incarnation of Vishnu
Deo — God
Ram + Deo = Ramdev
(Ram God)

The solution to this came at the end of the story I was related by the men: "He was buried here because he was holy,[15] and because he still performs miracles people come to him and call him Ram Deo and even *pir*."[16] Makkhanlal's formula and the legends that are related at the tomb allow the holiest of holies for Muslims, namely Mecca, to be brought together with the holiest of holies for Hindus, the god Ram, who is one of the incarnations of the supreme god Vishnu, in the name and being of the saint Ram Deo Pir. With that his holiness is not kept from anyone, so that everybody, whether of a high or low caste, or from the Muslim groups or the Indian scheduled tribes,[17] can find their way to him by making him their *una catholicam ecclesiam* which both brings together and heals.

Bhanabhai's temple is such a place. He sits before Ram Deo Pir's picture. Flowers and four green animals made of cloth have been placed at the *pir's* feet.[18] Rising above them is incense. Sitting behind Bhanabhai is his assistant, and behind them the congregation. Bhanabhai is small and delicately built, and modest by nature. The people address him with "Babu". They bring their complaints to him. "My wife has left me", says one man, "my cow has disappeared," says another, and "I still have no children," says a woman. "Have you obeyed Ram Deo Pir?" Babu replies to the first, "Have you sacrificed a cockerel?" he asks the next, and "Have you fasted?" he asks the woman. And thus the universal theatre which is staged at all times by sufferers and healers the world over likewise takes place here. The sufferer talks about his complaints, the healer says what they are and where they come from. The sufferer does more: He confesses in both meanings of the term. And from the healer he receives the word that will create order, the word that upholds the client, gives him a hold and allows him to act once again — so that soon he will fare better. Bhanabhai sits before his god, his saint. He acts eye to eye with him.

"What is going on between the two of them is beyond your comprehension in Europe," says Vikram Nath. "It sometimes takes just a fraction of a second, but it gives you power, a power that cannot be described but which you can take with you, back to your home, for instance. For us Hindus and Jains[19] the representation of a saint is also the saint himself. Perhaps it's the same for you with the communion wafer which stands for Jesus," he adds.

We should recall here the pilgrim who fell into a deep rapture and trance before the mountain god Golu when looking at him in his shrine; here too the state was triggered by face-to-face contact. And we can also recall the gaze of the actor in the Hindi film, of the protagonist of good, say, and what the spectator feels that this triggers inside him.

Bhanabhai's temple is a place of congregation for low-caste Hindus, but members of other religions, such as Muslims, also take part, as well as the people from the surrounding tribal districts. They maintain this centre through their presence, their devotion. These are people who do not visit the temples of orthodox Hinduism or of the established gods. As we left we heard the rhyming dialogue that went on constantly between Babu and the people seeking help gradually fading behind us:

Help-seeker: My whole body is trembling, my skin is also burning, I'm afraid that I am possessed by...

Babu: No, don't worry, there is nothing right now...

Help-seeker: ... by a nasty...

Babu: ... that's simply life, don't think about it any more...

Help-seeker: ... evil spirit because the cow's also gone...

Babu (in nasal sing-song voice): And if that's the case, then take the cockerel and sacrifice it to Ramdeopir, then it will all be alright, then...

Later that day we asked him what had prompted him to do what he now does. He told us of how his son had fallen ill, and how he had taken the matter into his own hands. He had taken his son to a guru who was a devotee of Ram Deo Pir and who helped him after going into trance. In that way they had healed his son. He had remained afterwards with the guru as his apprentice, and later the guru personally installed him here. He experienced his first trance on his own, here in his home. It is this trance in which he tries to give those seeking help the right answers to their life crises. He has also learned to dispense healing herbs and thus provide alleviation to physical suffering, which makes him a healer.

We drove back to the town where we heard of a Muslim who has already nominated himself a *pir* although he is still alive, calling himself Pir Zada Hafiz Sayed Mehfozali Aqadri in full. The name indicates great superiority. *Pirs* are the holy Muslims, and *sayeds* those who can trace their origins back to the circles of the prophet. And Pir Zada Hafiz is also a man of the word, of the intellect. He says that he collaborates with the municipal hospital, for he often sends cases there. He does not want to have anything to do with spirits and their mediums and trance, rather he wants to keep them at bay from his world. He does not get involved with things like that, that's not done any more, he says. His practice is full. His name is widely known and his therapeutic procedures are comprehensible to his patients. So they come to him with all their physical and non-physical ailments and he treats them with words from the Koran. If the patient's sufferings are of a supernatural origin, he places a text that he has selected in an amulet and recommends the patient to wear it. If the ailments are of a physical nature he takes the yellow pigment of saffrons, writes with this a sura from the Koran on a piece of paper, and then at once immerses the paper in water and hands the concoction to the patient as a healing draught. The clear distinction between these two approaches is matched by the clear success of his practice. He does not take anything from the people who visit him, unless, he admits, they want to make a donation. He would be willing to accept a donation.

We leave the orderly world of the *pir* and carry on through the town, which is full. Endless crowds of people surge like waves through the main streets, the men mostly dressed in white shirts, often with *dhotis*,[20] but also sometimes with trousers, the women in brightly coloured saris or *salwar* and *kamis*.[21] "Where do they all come from?" I wonder. "This stream of people must come to an end some time, or at least diminish. At night, perhaps?" A medical institution catches my eye, and

I point a questioning finger at a sign depicting two large and two little people with a text beneath which could roughly be translated as: "Two children alone make a happy home." "We're not going there," says Vikram Nath, "or are you about to get interested in politics?"

It is the India of Indira Gandhi and her "emergency laws" that is represented here.[22] I continue on my way, astonished at the contradictions. These crowds of people and the ruthless machinations of family planning politics were a dangerous mixture during that epoch, and their products a crime. Yet even I, a mere traveller, am unsettled by the stream of people here in the town, a stream that is so infinitely large and yet quite normal.

In town we are told about a man who bears the title *Chaus Rifai* and describes himself as a fakir. He had been given the title by the head of a Muslim order of monks, and it indicates that he possesses abilities that stretch beyond the social and everyday world. We go and look for him and find a very easy-going man whose rounded constitution radiates calm, to us at least, and presumably to those who bring him their sufferings, for his waiting room is already full, full of women. We are asked in and find him seated cross-legged on a mat in front of a woman and reading out a text. We have walked in on an action which he has staged in order to heal this woman. We sit down very quietly at the side of the room.

The woman is sitting on a black cloth, on which white flowers and *urad* beans (*phaseolus mungo*) have been scattered, and has spread a white cloth over herself. In front of her is a bottle to which she is linked several times over in a mysterious manner by a length of string; she looks at it with a strained expression while the *chaus* reads. The two of them can hardly be seen. The incense billows up in the room and makes the people appear like shades. On closer inspection we can see how the string connects the woman to the bottle; it runs from out of the bottle to her foot, encircles her large toe and then passes up to her pelvis where it disappears under her clothes, only to first reappear by her face. There it travels up over her right ear and then between her lips to her other ear, and from there back down to the neck of the bottle. I try to picture to myself how the *chaus* could have attached the string to her without infringing the bounds of decency. He now tells the woman to inhale the smoke that is issuing from the small piece of incense (*resina benzoe*).[23] His voice grows quieter as she breathes. After a good thirty minutes the *chaus* undoes the lengths of string that link the woman with the bottle. She straightens herself up. He blows at her across the text he had been reading and then inserts the piece of paper with the text into a small bottle, stoppers it and hands it to the already departing woman.

He turns to us without any sign of surprise. "She was ill for a long time," he says, "heart and stomach problems. She couldn't have been cured without a doctor, and now she comes to me. If you like you can stay and watch me while I work."

While he is still talking the next woman comes in and sits on the place her predecessor has vacated. She has brought a bottle of water which she hands to the *chaus*. "Which spring is the water from?" he asks. She gives three names. He says that the springs are good and that the water has what he requires for his work. But now he only reads one text — sometimes he reads several — while blowing into the bottle, which he then returns to the woman. She now asks him for the written text as well, so that she can put it in the bottle with the water which he said was good and healing, and allow it, too, to act on her. The *chaus* is reluctant to agree and explains that she does not require it, but then he relents and the woman leaves the room with her bottle under her arm.

When the next customer arrives I am almost able to satisfy my curiosity about how he manages to thread the strings. The woman silently follows the example of her predecessor and sits down before the fakir. She has brought much more with her than the others. A *seer*, the equivalent of almost two pounds, of mung beans, blossoms, six yards of black cloth, a piece of *loban* (incense), a white cloth, a reel of cotton and a large bottle of water. She hands them all to the fakir. Without saying a word he spreads out the black cloth, arranges the blossoms and mung beans on it and indicates that the waiting woman should now lie down on it. He sweeps a switch of peacock feathers up and down the length of her body, and while he does this the woman lowers herself slowly and silently on to the cloth that the *chaus* has prepared for her. The healer lets her take her time, but he fills up the passing minutes by placing the bottle at her feet, inserting the end of the cotton into its neck and drawing the thread along her body: up along her leg from her foot, where he makes the first loop, along her thigh, where he places the thread under her blouse, which reaches down to her knee, from whence he pushes it up along her upper body to her shoulder where he fastens it once more. Just how was obscured though in the vital moment by the thick clouds of smoke from the incense. When he reaches the woman's head, he passes the thread up over her forehead to the top of her head before returning it to the bottle, into which he inserts it once again.

The woman lies there tensely before him. When the lump of *loban* is lit and he blows the smoke over her she disappears momentarily amidst a cloud of smoke, so that her presence can only be discerned by her short choking cough. Now he, her healer, gets to business and reads her text to her. This, together with the water, the incense and the blossoms and beans on the cloth, is supposed to heal her.

Later, as evening draws in and the waiting room empties, we ask him: "What does the healing? And where do all the things that you require to heal others come from?" He knows exactly and gives us the list that we want.

He was very young and had no one to help him because he had no more family. So he trained as a healer and received the healing power from his teacher, a man who accepts pupils and hands on the power and knowledge he possesses. They learned about health and illness from him, but the actual healing power only came at the end. It is transmitted to the pupil during a ceremony that also marks the end of the training. "And then there's the water," he continues. "If the water is good and from the right place it has healing powers. It removes the ailments and the sickness from your body. If you drink it, of course, but also through the threads that link the water with the patient's body. It draws out the illness, one can see how this happens if one examines the bottle directly after the session with the patient. One can see particles in the water that weren't there before. And then there's the smoke which, although it purifies, does not directly heal. I also use texts, specific ones for each illness, no, not every illness, rather for each part of the body, for your heart, your head, your stomach or what have you. I blow this text into the water for the patient and then hand them the water. The text is in it so that it will carry on working."

The day had been a long one. We leave, impressed by the genealogies of health-giving and -taking: Ram Deo Pir, whose healing power still works centuries after his death, the word of the Koran, the water from the springs. But we are even more impressed by the situations that are staged to heal the sick and the methods the healers have thought up for allowing the energy they administer to flow into the patient: from bottles via threads into and back out of the body, via peacock feathers, beans and blossoms, via the written word, words blown into the air or immersed in water, and the word of Babu spoken from the world of trance. It appeared that, once they had initially opened themselves to a source of the sacred and healing, the people here could accept every course that is taken by the healing force. And the power which seemed to heal uses every such course, like the water in a rough river.

We are both feeling tired. The *chaus* has advised us to spend the night in the guest house of the Janata Party.[24] "Mostly there's somewhere you can stay," he adds. We find the house and ask the cook whether he would allow us to sleep in the house. Two rooms or two beds would be good. "There's nothing free," comes the reply. Vikram Nath hands him ten rupees and the cook takes us to two rooms behind the kitchen. They are empty, which is just fine with us after a day so full of people and things, for there is nothing else that I want now than this iron bedstead with its lumpy mattress, the bucket of water in the corner with the small hole in the wall to allow the used water to flow away, and the light bulb on the naked wall so that I can jot down a few notes. The lumps in the mattress are hard and one must first find the lay of the land before one can get to sleep. Then, as I turn off the light, I see two eyes staring through the grille in front of the window.

I am unable to decide whether this is a dream that is showing me one, just one, of the many, often gaping pairs of eyes from the day gone by, or whether the gaze is here in this very moment. I drag two sections of an old screen in front of the window and put off the decision till tomorrow. And the next morning it becomes easier because now the sun is shining through the screen and I can see the body of this pair of eyes outside the window: a silver langur monkey, a female who expects that I will give her a little something. Which is precisely what happens, for there is no getting away from her gaze.

Vikram Nath is already sitting outside, waiting. I join him, accompanied by my notebook. He fills in the gaps in what I observed the day before, as well as in my prior knowledge. I write what I hear. And with that we are ready to set off again. We find another successful healer in the same town, a man who attracts hundreds of patients to his practice and cures their ails. He is also a specialist. Once the patient is in front of him he throws rice grains into the air which divine the person's health and mental state. If an uneven number of grains falls in front of him he takes on the case, because then it has a supernatural cause. Not that he could not resort to healing herbs for ailments with natural causes, such as *Coccina indica* when the women suffer from their special problems, but that is not his main interest, that is just a part of his metier, just as he has learned from the person who trained him. When the number of rice grains is uneven he must decide where the mischief comes from. Then Jivanji Rathod, who is a *lohar*[25] or smithy, must enter the darkness, into the realm of the unsatisfied ancestors (*pitu*) who are still attached to life, or even of the *jinn* or cemetery spirits[26] who live among the dead and seize what they lack from the living. And he will have to continue searching in this realm until he has found the cause and can act. He does this with texts and words. When it is a case of *jinn* that is draining the sick person's strength, he writes these words in saffron and milk on straw. The straw is immersed in water and the patient has to drink it over seven days. In other cases ink suffices for the text, which is likewise written on straw and handed to the patient in water to drink.

"How does this evil descend on the patient?" I now want to know, to which he answers:

"Anyone who deviates from the daily order, anyone who drops their guard, eats or says the wrong thing, and is perhaps also at the wrong place and with the wrong people, can be injured by the evil and dark forces from the other side. The *jinn*, the *pitu* are simply waiting for this and keep constant watch at particular spots, both in town and in the country. You can protect yourself you know, but you have to know how and what form the protection should take. That is particularly difficult," he continues, "when you have been lured and attacked by a *churäl*.[27] Suddenly you hear a lullaby, perhaps the very one your mother used to sing to you, which entices you and which you want to follow wherever it goes. *Churäls* are ghosts with a particular thirst for blood and bones, for life and limb. That's because they were formerly young women who died while they were pregnant — while carrying a life inside themselves. Thus they are dead two times over, and they're also the worst when it comes to exorcising them," he says ". And they keep luring people with lullabies which they never got to sing during their own lifetimes. And if you follow them you get ill. They enter your bones and your body, blood issues from your lungs and your stool and the doctors cannot find out what's causing it, and if it is a *churäl* they can't help you anyhow."

We leave Jivanji, who has explained to us his methods and the way he ascertains the truth during the pause between two consultations. His waiting room is full. Like the others we visited previously, he has a large circle of followers.

I jot down the word "sirens" and try to picture the lullaby and its sound. Is this sound that can draw you to your death metallic, or perhaps long and drawn-out, or is it sweet? And how does the man from the smithy, the *lohar* Jivanji, revert this reversal? What must the text, the word that he puts in the water to be drunken be like for it to change the direction that the *churäl* gives to those who listen? Jivanji searches for the words personally in Muslim and Hindu texts. Jivan, incidentally, means life in Hindi; *ji* is simply an honorific suffix.

It is noon. Vikram Nath has bought us bus tickets. We drive off into the mountains to the east of the town, to Ahwa. It is Holi, the spring festival of the Hindus. It is celebrated at full moon in the month of *Phalgun* (March). Anyone who has some red paint — symbol of blood and life — at hand and something to squirt it with can do everything that is normally not allowed: grab women by the hair, or under their saris, spray red-coloured water into their employer's face, hold up the bus on a country lane and demand money... At night Holi fires are lit at every cross-road. They are sacred because when the fire-goddess is worshipped and offerings are placed for her in the fire she will undo injuries and purify and heal. The villages to the east of Gujarat hold spring funfairs at Holi. But by the time we arrive at Ahwa it is already too late to visit the spring festival. As we walk the two kilometres to the fairground we meet all of the people who put on the festival returning from the other direction: the idol sellers, the confectionery vendors, the showmen, the stall owners.

We also encounter a small wooden temple borne on a palanquin. The bearers stop. They place the temple by the wayside and open the little door: a pair of fixed, staring eyes peer out of the small portable shrine. It is a goddess which is doing the staring and being carried around; she is wearing a kind of crown on her head and a sari round her body, and is brandishing a sabre or sword in one of her four hands. Who is she? It's the goddess Harai, they tell me, and they sell me an amulet from her. One of the shrine-carriers tells me that he also sometimes enters into trance when the goddess is inside him, and then he can heal with her aid: rabies and dog-bites and a few others things. The crowd is too large and they disappear among the seething mass before I can ask any more questions. Only later in the evening do I find the time to remove the wrapper from the amulet, which one is not supposed to do, and study it. I find the goddess who had stared at me from her little, wooden, house-like shrine; she has four arms and is sitting on an animal, a dog perhaps, or maybe a tiger. It could be Ambica, one of the three great goddesses of this region who is worshipped all over Gujarat, in which case her mount must be a tiger.

Later I find the clue that solves the question of the palanquin-occupant's identity: "*Hadkair* is the goddess who protects people from rabies", I read, and "since this illness is primarily contracted from dog-bites, *Hadkair* is generally depicted riding a dog" (Fischer, Jain and Shah, 1982). The authors continue, saying that in an emergency "... a person infected by rabies is brought before the goddess *Hadkair*. The sufferer promises not to eat any rice or sugar for one and a quarter months and to avoid coconuts and bathing for the duration. Nor should they eat any cold foods during this time.[28] The month of *Chaitra* (April) is considered particularly auspicious for honouring pledges of offerings. People maintain that even previously broken promises will be forgiven if one honours a vow to the goddess *Hadkair* during this period."

It is only just March, but perhaps it is already an auspicious time to meet the goddess and gain her help against sickness and evil. Reading on, the authors say: "Some municipal hospitals have small shrines where the patients can worship the goddess while waiting for the doctor." They hire welfare and well-being, worship the bringers of this grace, disseminate it, transport, speak and when in trance dance it, I reflect, while toying with *Hadkair*'s image between my fingers.

Wherever we go we find cures being staged, as if on this journey we were following a choreography of healing that is invisible to us, within the gradually emerging topography of the paths to the healers, to the power and healing that they bestow. It is dark so we hurry with the rest back to the village of Ahwa. There is nowhere to stay there except for a small pilgrims' camp. The administrator gives me his bed which I share with his wife and three small children. I accept gratefully and fall asleep before I have time to check what I suspect.

The next morning I wake up with a cruel itching. Although *Hadkair*, whose amulet was lying beside me in bed, had protected me from dog-bites, she had overlooked the dog's inhabitants, the fleas. I ask for a bucket of water and a secluded corner of the grounds. As I remove my clothes more fleas jump off of me than I count. I can count the bites though: 75. I shall have to ask *Hadkair* to enlarge her repertoire if I ever get the opportunity to meet her again: "Dear *Hadkair*, please keep the fleas, or at least any quantity of fleas numbering more than three, away from me because for God's, or rather the Goddess's sake I can't go on travelling like this!"

We carry on and visit the neighbouring villages. While Vikram Nath inquires about healers and temples that contain healing deities, I look for buildings in which the night can be spent uncontested. Neither of us finds what we are looking for, so we carry on till we reach a bus stop from which we travel that same night to Surat, the largest harbour of the Mughal dynasty, as well as of the slave age and the textile trading age, until the role was taken over by Mumbai under the British during the "Company Bahadur" age.[29] We have no difficulty finding a hotel near the bus terminus, which is convenient because we want to continue our journey first thing the next morning. The early sunrise greets us with the siren-like voice of a *shehnai* (oboe) pursued by a tabla which wafts through the rooms of the hotel. Then a voice joins in. I am still not awake and think there must be a *churäl* under my bed. *That* wakes me up in no time! A sweet, tender, tempting woman's voice sings: "How shall I tell you, that you live in my heart, mere dill me, mere dill me, *rehte ho... dill me*," and still echoes after us as we walk to the bus stop. Just harmless Hindi film music. Everyone knows the film, the melody and the text that is blaring out of the speakers, everyone knows the plot it refers to and consequently finds themselves, acoustically at first, in a kind of invisible community which unites all who follow these sounds and can associate with their images.[30]

It is still very early and we find a seat on the bus immediately. The journey is long and hot. We have to change several times and we still have not had any breakfast. We pass through Baroda, the beautiful town renowned for its art and university, but today we simply change there. The train is small, just five carriages and all with wooden benches. It chugs along slowly, we need two hours for just thirty kilometres. We are travelling to Pavagadh, which has a mountain on which the great goddess *Maha Kali*, who reputedly has a chain of human heads about her neck and rides a tiger, has her home. The train stops again, this time in a hamlet whose station consists of nothing more than a row of wooden planks. Our nap comes to a sudden end. People board, mount, jump on, climb on to and clamber over the train from all quarters. There is nowhere left to sit. Or lie, for the luggage racks above us are suddenly full of reclining travellers. The compartment seems full, but that does not stop them. I crane my neck out of the window and look up between the dangling legs outside to a roof overcrowded with people. The train has become a human beehive that has been captured by a swarm. Silver jewellery sparkles from arms and legs and ears and sometimes even noses, and jingles quietly but perpetually all around our compartment — from the floor to the luggage rack — to the accompaniment of the customary noises that had enveloped us in our asleep. The women are wrapped in printed saris, mostly in red. Often one can see only the heavy silver bangles on their feet and hands, and then brief flashes of faces decorated with small, bluish-black tattoos. The men have impressive moustaches and mostly a white turban perched on their heads. Their clothes consist of a shirt and a white dhoti. "What are you people?" I mumble to the nearest face which is just a breath away. "We are Katolia *Rajputs*," says the face under the turban next to me. They are *Rathvas*, Vikram Nath scribbles to me on a piece of paper. He chose this form of communication in order to avoid any dispute.[31] "And where are you all travelling to?" I continue. "Mela, mela," some ten or twenty faces reply, "we're going to a fair,[32] which is not too far now." And the fair-goers dismount the train in a small station no larger than the one in which they had boarded.

I am sucked along in their wake. I disboard, much to the astonishment of Vikram Nath, who wants to travel to Pavagadh to the mother goddess Kali. But we follow the fair-goers and after less than two hours reach the fair in full swing at around noon. Behind a longish row of stalls lined up before a hill we can see two ferris wheels in motion, each with four rocking, swinging gondolas containing brightly-clad visitors who are singing for sheer joy. We follow the procession of people, and purchase sweets from the candy vendors and "koldringkoldring" (cold drinks) from the drink sellers.

Then we see six youths coming down from the village, whose torsos are bare and painted completely in yellow *(haldi)*.[33] They are walking along beneath a white cloth canopy that is supported by four men wearing turbans and shirts. The youths' beautiful bodies glisten and are clad only in *dhotis*. They keep their gazes directed slightly downwards as they walk on over the curve of the hill, each with a coconut in his hands.[34] "Where are they off to?" I ask the man nearest to me. "To the fire goddess," he replies, "in order to honour the vows they made for their recuperation." And before there is any more time for questions, the next group passes by. Their canopy is red. They can already be seen far away on the crest of the hill, as they march along beneath the tall trees. Once again the pilgrims' bodies are completely coated in turmeric, which is always regarded as a cure-all in India. The bodies of these singing youths have been carefully oiled all over, as has their hair. They are escorted along the wayside by young women who are singing and dressed completely in red. And now the next canopy is slowly being brought down the hill, and this time there are also women beneath it. But only men do the carrying, and they too are singing.

It could also be a wedding procession, I think, like those of the *Rathvas* described by Jyotindra Jain:

"On the day of the wedding, independently at the houses of the bride and the groom, a ritual of symbolically grinding paddy takes place. The paddy is suspended in a piece of cloth and held over the heads of the bride and the groom. After this, *pithi*, a paste of turmeric powder, oil, some flour, camphor etc. is applied to the bodies of the marital couple... When the wedding booth is set up, a pot filled with water topped by a coconut is placed inside." (Jain, 1984)

I ask once again. "No, they are going to the fire goddess,

not to a wedding," I am told, and the person who replies takes me by the hand and leads me there.

"We have to fast the night before," my companion tells me, "when we are going to honour a vow we made the year before. The vow goes as follows," he says. "I shall walk over burning coals on the second day of Holi if I overcome the illness that is now in my body." The young men who had paraded past us with their bodies painted with *haldi* (turmeric) have come to make their offerings here because, thanks to the goddess, their bodies have overcome their illnesses.

As we arrive at the site of the fire below we see that the young men have stepped out from under the baldachin-like canopy, which has been laid to one side. A gateway of sugarcanes and mango leaves has been erected before the glowing field of coals. The young men have now covered their heads. One man stands at the front of them, holding a round, shiny metal tray in his hand which he keeps moving in a circle. Standing on the tray, which is called a *thali*,[35] is a small oil lamp, some red powder and rice. The man is performing a particular kind of *puja*,[36] an act of worship termed *arti*,[37] in preparation for the fire offering. All those who are about to walk over the coals now also perform *arti*, moving the oil lamp in a circle before their covered faces. They stand in groups and wait until the lamp is passed to them. Set to the right of the gateway is a sword, and to the left is an iron bar. "The fire was already lit this morning," someone says, "by a *Tadvi*[38] who does it every year. He takes twigs and places leaves on top of them and then lights the fire and tends it for an hour."

The coal-walking can now begin. Everyone, almost all of the people who have come to the fire, have done their worship, honoured their vow, and made an offering of a coconut or a little money. Then the man who is performing the *arti* begins to shake violently. He holds a bird in one hand which he first prays to and immediately after sacrifices. And in precisely this moment his body is seized by trance. He walks across the coals, the bird still in his hand, then he returns to the entrance, places the bird with the other offerings, takes the sword, prays to the fire and circles it several times so as to inaugurate it for the pilgrims. Prior to this leaves from the *neem* tree are placed on the coals.[39]

Fresh leaves are placed on the coals for each fire-walker. They are also used as a remedy for skin diseases, stomach complaints and cramps. Now the pilgrims set out one after the other: first through the gateway of leaves that leads to the fire and then through a second gateway that opens on to the glowing coals. They walk over the embers with quick, but not hasty, steps and at the end sink their feet with ashes still clinging to them into a large heap of dark green cow dung that is situated at the far end of the walk. Finally each must pass through a last gateway made of twigs and leaves before returning to the everyday world. The fire walkers, who have put their own bodies through fire in order to honour the vows they made in order to be healed, disappear among the alleys between the stalls of the *mela*. Their bodies are considered to have been purified after walking over the coals.

This event, which the *Rathvas* hold once a year to mark the restoration of their health, is the most impressive staging of healing that I have seen. The overcoming of their anxieties and pain, the presence of the divine and the acting out of a fundamental trust when the vow-taker's feet touch the coals, amounts to an accumulation of healing factors that far outdoes anything that we had previously encountered.

"The fire," I was later told by a man who had fire-walked here in the West, "continued to fill me with energy for days after, indeed it healed me of all of my complaints. I entered a different reality, that of fire, which seemed cool to my feet."

The Tadvi who laid the fire says that his people have been doing this now for seven generations and that previously they were *Rathvas*, one of the tribal groups. But now they have based their income on agriculture and they are called Tadvi. He shows us his house where we are greeted with tea and shade, a true delight in this intense heat which causes the air shimmer. We sit on a mat. The Tadvi, whose name is Kalabhai, tells us once again that what we have seen has been performed in this village for seven generations. Painted on the walls of this room, which also houses a large wickerwork grain container, are horses, lots and lots of horses. They are running from the left to the right, mounted and unmounted. Some are copulating with other animals, even though they are mounted. One is copulating with a woman and yet has a saddle on its back. Further to the front of the procession a king with a sword can be seen riding a horse, followed by a woman who is also on horseback and between them a bird. "Those are *Pithoro* and *Pithori* during their wedding procession," Kalbhai tells us, "the bird is the black cuckoo. We believe that it is *Pithori*'s mother."

Jain writes on this: "Pithoro is one of the most respected gods of the *Rathvas*. He is a god connected with the household as well as the welfare of cattle. Every *Rathva* family desires *Pithoro*'s presence in the house for protection and welfare." Pithoro is the nephew of *Babo Ind*, and Jyotindra Jain also writes in his book *Painted Myths of Creation* that the *Rathvas* have kept up the ancient Indian cult of the Vedic God *Indra* in the form of this uncle, Babo Ind. The *Rathvas* paint the creation of their world once or twice a year on the walls of their houses, which makes them into temples (Jain, 1984, pp.18 and 61ff).

"And what about the fire that you walk across," we ask, "and the sword and the bird?" "That is the sword of Pithoro, which frees the way to the fire. The bird must be sacrificed. It is the spirit of the bride's mother. It is called *Kali Koyal*, the black cuckoo. She makes space for the fire, but simultaneously holds it in check. Thus the fire remains small and on the place foreseen for it," the Tadvi answers.

We thank him for the shade and his hospitality and then leave, because it will take us quite a while to reach the small railway station. But it takes even longer for us to emerge from the reality of the *Rathvas* and to link it with what we have assigned ourselves, a field research trip.

"So what are we going to do now?" I ask Vikram Nath as the small train slowly enters Baroda. But he never listens to me when he has a wad of *pan* in his cheek. That is *his* time, I should know that by now. Probably we will travel to the grave of the Muslim saint whose "outpost" we had visited in Mumbai. It is supposed to exert a great attraction on sick people whose illnesses cannot be identified.

NOTES

1. The life energy *num*, as understood by the !Kung San, is comparable to the Indian concept of *prana*. *Num* has its seat at the base of the spine, and when it rises it produces *Kia*, an ecstatic state (Katz, 1985).
2. Obeyesekere points in his article "Depression, Buddhism, and the Work of Culture" (1985) to the interaction between the culture of medicine and the diagnosis of depression. Feelings or affects lack the dimension of space in our Western culture of rationalisation and rationality, he writes, and thus are conceptualised as illnesses, as is the case of depression. In a society though that lives according to Buddhist precepts, as for instance in Sri Lanka, hopelessness is not a spaceless concept that has to be categorised as an illness. Rather it is one of the basic assumptions of Buddhist society that life is concerned with despair and its mastery, and that this is "normal". If one pursues this line of thought it becomes clear that the export and clinical realization of Western psychiatric concepts, whether of depression or anything else, amounts to cultural colonialism. Thus Obeyesekere is a teacher for all who wish to learn to really "read".
3. *Bopa* is the term in northern India for a possession specialist. Every India settlement has its *bopas*, who are generally members of the lower castes. They have one or more deities who will who enter their bodies and possess them when summoned in order to assist them in the process of healing clients.
4. *Ganesha* or *Ganesh* is the elephant-headed son of the deity Shiva and his wife Parvati. According to a post-Vedic myth he is solely the son of Parvati, who created him by means of parthenogenesis: he came to life from the water with which Parvati washed herself after she had made love to Shiva (O'Flaherty, 1980). Shiva later decapitated Parvati's son in a fit of conjugal jealousy, but immediately after provided him with an elephant's head that happened to be at hand (ibid.). According to other sources, the elephant-headed deity originates from tribal cultures that have been "incorporated" into Hinduism. Ganesh is often portrayed in Gujarat in embroideries and fabric prints.
5. The book (B.Pfleiderer and L.Lutze, 1985) comprises a collection of articles by Indian writers and journalists, as well

as works by the editors on the role of film in present-day Indian society.

6. *Bombaihindipilum* is a Hindi film produced in Mumbai. "Philum" is the frequently encountered pronunciation of the English word "film".
7. *Dargah Sharif* is the term for Muslim centres of pilgrimage in India. In this case it refers to the martyr Mira Datar who is defined as such by a legend. *Sayed* is a title used among Indian Muslims to denote that someone is of Arab origin but is not directly descended from Ali, the Prophet's son-in-law. The use of Ali as a first name suggests this line of descent. *Dargah* by itself means court and *sharif* means holy.
8. *Mujawar* literally means guide. Here it refers to the dignitaries of the shrine who impart the centre's sacred power to the pilgrims by such means as water, peacock feathers and cloth horses, as well as by circumambulation.
9. *Sawwali* literally means a questioner, one who comes with a question; here it refers to the pilgrims who find themselves caught up in a problem from which they hope to disentangle themselves at the shrine.
10. *Dupatta* is the cloth veil that is worn with the trouser suit called *salwar-kamis* or simply Punjabi dress.
11. *Chilla* denotes a place of pilgrimage that is derived from another, more importance centre. Here it is used to denote all of the personal, "satellite" Mira Datar Dargahs that have been erected by pilgrims to the main shrine, after bringing a "foundation" stone from the main centre at Unava, Gujarat. It is as it were a "genetic" designation or simply a place of remembrance.
12. *Hajri* is the Hindi or Urdu word for presence. It is used when the body has entered into a trance and a deity or spirit is assumed to be present within it. A body that is in *hajri* is possessed by another being. This possession is the prerequisite for *hajri*.
13. While *hajri* is primarily experienced by women, and is very often accompanied by much noise and activity, *ghum hajri* is a quiet form of trance which is often unaccompanied by any physical signs. Generally it is the men who say that they have been in *ghum hajri*. After speaking with those who have experienced it, one quickly gains the impression that this quiet trance is the "more distinguished" version of the same behaviour.

14. The neem tree *(Melia azederachi)* can be found at many north Indian shrines, both Muslim and Hindu. In the West it known by a variety of names, such as the chinaberry, Pride-of-India, or false sycamore, but most commonly as the margosa. It is related to the elder.
15. Although Hindus normally burn their dead, there are exceptions to this. Holy men, such as sadhus, are buried, as are pregnant women and *hijras* — the eunuchs and transvestites. The additional fact that Ram Deo Pir was buried makes even more of an exception and indeed a saint of him. Muslims always bury their dead, without exception. The Parsis lay their dead out for birds of prey to devour, and this is also sometimes done with transvestites. All those who are not to be cremated, with the exception of Parsis and transvestites, can also be committed to the waters of the Ganges.
16. *Pir* designates a Muslim saint in India. In the case of Ram Deo Pir we are looking at a syncretic phenomenon, because here elements of the Muslim faith are to be found in a Hindu shrine. The saint was a Hindu but nevertheless bore the additional title *pir* because he was also a member of the Muslim community.
17. A 50- to 60-million strong section of the Indian population consists of "tribals". In Gujarat these include the Bhils, the *Rathvas* and the Meghwals, to name just a few. The British introduced the term "scheduled tribes". This group is located at the lower end of the Hindu caste continuum. The British used these terms and categorisations to regulate the interactions between the individual Hindu groups. In this case the categorisation was to be accompanied by the granting of certain rights that would improve their lot.
18. Green is the colour of Islam.
19. Hindus and Jains worship their deities through the mediation of images. Thus they worship the deity through or by means of his image. Image worship of this kind is unknown in Islam. For this reason temples that have been the particular object of Muslim aggression have often been robbed of their images.
20. *Dhoti* denotes the white loincloth worn by men in rural districts.
21. *Salwar-kamis* is generally worn by women originating from the Punjab, hence the common name 'Punjabi dress'. Nowadays it is worn mostly by young girls in the north, while adult women wear the traditional sari.

22. The emergency laws were introduced during the latter half of the seventies by Indira Gandhi in order to protect her leadership. During her rule she introduced with the assistance of her son Sanjay Gandhi a somewhat militaristic family planning programme that had an intimidating effect on the populace.
23. The piece of *resina benzoe*, which is referred to there as *loban* and which we term incense, is used by many healing authorities in the area we visited as a means for exorcising evil spirits from the bodies of the possessed.
24. The Janata Party succeeded the Congress Party under Indira Gandhi at the end of the 1970s for a period of some three years.
25. The *lohars* are members of the very low caste of smiths. As in many other cultures, the smiths are often attributed with supernatural abilities. Traditionally the smiths lived in or beneath the black iron carts in which they travel from village to village and town to town. According to one legend, when Chittor, a mediaeval fort in Rajasthan, fell to Islamic invaders the *lohars* swore never to live in fixed abodes before the fort was freed of Muslims. The *lohars'* carts can still be seen all over northern India.
26. *Jinn* (or *jinnat* in the Arab plural) are spirits that dwell in the ground as well as frequently in graveyards. Often people would talk of *jinn* in cases of possession, for although they originate from the Arabic-Persian region, they are no less talked about by the Hindus. The jinn are viewed in the Near East as a pre-Arabic phenomenon.
27. A *churäl* is a female ghost. She is the product of a "nasty", which is to say unnatural death and is thus regarded as especially malevolent. Exorcising a *churäl* is considered to be particularly difficult.
28. In the whole of Asia, as well as incidentally in Latin America, all foodstuffs are placed within the schema of hot—cold, although this varies considerably from one location to the next. Thus mangoes are hot in one place and cold in another. Alcohol and meat are always viewed though as hot. In ayurvedic medicine certain ailments are regarded as the product of too much "hot" food, and others as the product of too much "cold". Dietetics and the bodily schema are viewed as in constant interplay, under the dominion of hot and cold substances. Consequently great attention has to be paid in

such countries to what is imbibed.

29. The unofficial rulership of the British before the declaration of the Empire was termed by the Indians "Company Bahadur".
30. The enormous popularity of the Hindi movie has led to the creation of a pan-Indian community of film-goers whose clothing, behaviour and everyday speech is influenced by the dialogues, the hit songs and the leading stars of the most celebrated films, and who constantly imitate the world of film. The culture in India is thus partly popular film culture, and likewise the film culture is popular everyday culture (see Pfleiderer and Lutze, 1985).
31. There is a tendency within the Indian caste system for an entire caste to strive for upward mobility. When for instance a caste assigned to the Shudras — the low-caste labourers — decides to ascend the social scale, it first assumes the caste denomination it aspires to, then its religious practices, and finally its day-to-day behaviour. In the state of Ahmedabad there are for example countless darzis — tailors — who suddenly gave themselves the surname Singh. A person named Singh is, however, a Kshatriya, a noble and member of the landowner caste, assuming he is not a Sikh. Much the same applies to the "tribals". When encountered in Gujarat or Rajasthan, they will say "we are Rajputs", i.e. Rajasthani Kshatriyas. In order to avoid casting open doubt on these claims, Vikram Nath wrote the answer down on paper.
32. *Mela* is translated in the English ethnographic literature as fair or festival. The *melas* described in this chapter are the festivals that are held in this region by the indigenous populace before, during and after the spring festival of Holi.
33. *Haldi* is a yellow paste or powder made from turmeric. The paste is used to heal wounds, and the yellow powder is used ritually in numerous cults. It can be found in every Indian home pharmacy.
34. The coconut, which is used in numerous rituals, is viewed as a substitute for the human sacrifices previously made to the female deity.
35. A *thali* is a round metal plate with a raised rim that is used for eating meals. In addition, it is used for offering food or other substances to the deities in their temples.
36. The ritual veneration of deities is called a *puja*, and the ritual

expert or assistant a *pujari*.

37. The act of circling lit candles or oil lamps before an idol or the representation of a deity is referred to as *arti*.
38. The *Tadvis* (pronounced talvis) are a sub-group of the *Rathvas*, a tribe of central India.
39. cf. note 14.

Chapter 4

Mira Datar Dargah

Arrival

We have travelled via Ahmedabad, where we visited Hiranand and his wife, who shared our astonishment at what we had to tell from our travels. But we also received plenty of advice and helpful explanations, for they are both ethnographers and know the region. They have introduced us to Anil who has places himself and his car at our disposal for the day in order to take us to the small district town of Unava north of Mehasana. We eagerly accept his offer because the car will take us to our destination in just two hours, instead of the whole day it would have taken us by bus and train.

If one travels from Ahmedabad along the highway to the north-east across the fertile plains of Gujarat, one arrives on the south side of the small town of Unava. If one arrives by the noonday bus, as we often did once we had started working there, one finds the place cloaked in that typical pall of silence that can be found all over India during the intense midday heat. The water buffalos have gone to the temple pond in search of coolness: only their nostrils are visible, even their eyes are submerged; dogs have stretched out in the shade and grown motionless; the goats have moved on from removing the banana-skins and other scraps from the streets to calm rumination.

The dust sent up by our car sinks to reveal an empty, deserted, village street. The water in the pond is smooth and reflects the haze of the midday sky. The dealers, whose wooden booths line the entrance to the shrine, the main shrine of the Mira Datar Dargah pilgrimage centre, are taking a midday nap on or under their counters. Even the numbers of the inevitable hordes of children who normally beleaguer the strangers with their questions have been decimated at this hour.

A representative of the shrine authorities who keeps an eye on all the new arrivals — whether by bus, rickshaw or car — in order to establish contact with the pilgrims as they arrived, steps from the shade of a street restaurant and slowly approaches us.

This scene will be repeated, year after year, for as long as we "gather data" here and conduct our "field research". For a number of years I set off each spring to India during the university vacations in order to conduct interviews here with the women who purport to be possessed by nasty spirits, and consequently have to scream wildly and roll about in the dust in front of the tomb of Saint Mira Datar and pray for relief.

"Back again? How long will you be staying this time?" comes the familiar question from the man who refers to himself as a *mujawar*, which means roughly a guide to the shrine. Later on he will ask after my companions from the previous year, Dr. Hans and Dr. Irmtraud, for instance, a couple of interested doctors who once accompanied me with the aim of getting to know trance from their own psychiatric standpoint. Or my students who made tape recordings for their theses. And then he will tell me about the changes or their renewed troubles with the local authorities over the sanitary installations, which can never be good enough.

But on this occasion, on our first arrival, he merely introduces himself: "I am Muhammadhusen. Follow me! I shall show you the shrine of Saint Mira Datar."

As he makes his way to the shrine, the pilgrim can already see in the distance the gentle movement of the flag on top of the tower that they call the *sulli*. The flag is green, the colour of the prophet, and tells the pilgrim that he or she is expected. The court of the saint, which is called the *darbar* or *dargah*, the royal court, is ready to receive visitors.

"We have roughly sixty *mujawars*," Muhammadhusen tells

us, "who work for the *sawwalis*, the pilgrims, wait for them and accompany during their stay. They are all descendants of the saint's brother, so they are all members of his family."

We approach the entrance. The small number of shoes at the feet of the slumbering shoe attendant reveals that only a handful of visitors has arrived. I buy some rose petals and a bangle from a stall close to the entrance and, in keeping with the custom, allow myself to be led to the saint's tomb by my *mujawar*. As is the case with all women, I am not allowed to enter the interior of the tomb complex and have to be represented there by my *mujawar*. After a prayer to saint Sayed 'Ali Mira Datar, he places my rose petals on the red and green shroud, which he calls a *gilaf*, together with the bangle which he subsequently returns to me. The bangle now has something of the quality radiated by the tomb. This quality, which is used here as a healing power, is called *karamat*. It will benefit anyone who wears the bangle.

I remain standing in the women's courtyard. A number of women is sitting on the ground reading from the Koran. They mutter softly and quickly while swaying their hips. Before them is a long row of graves which is separated by marble walls. These are the final resting places of the saint's numerous relatives. It is through them that the *mujawars* trace their kinship to the saint. Other women are lying on the ground under their headscarfs — exhausted, perhaps after a morning spent in trance, which everyone here calls *hajri*. The women's courtyard is partly roofed over, partly walled in, and partly exposed. It is situated on the east side of the complex. On the opposite side is the men's courtyard. On the west side. And the west is the direction of Mecca. That is the better side.

The men sit on the ground of the courtyard, leaning against the projections from the wall. Some are muttering almost inaudibly while at the same time allowing their strings of small wooden beads to run automatically through their fingers. Behind the men's courtyard are the public sleeping quarters for the "lowlier" male visitors. Inside a walled-in enclosure to the north is the white distempered mosque, and before that a neat, empty courtyard. The entire tomb complex is surrounded by quarters for the pilgrims — small, dark rooms with no windows, which house entire families. At the moment, midday, the majority of the narrow wooden doors have been chained shut: the inhabitants are resting after the morning's rituals and daily duties.

Even the administrative offices of the *mujawars*, who otherwise are constantly bent over their account books, or sending prayer postcards to former pilgrims, or checking through their address lists, even these rooms are quiet during the midday hours. The guardians of the shrine and its healing power have gone home to lunch with their families who live in the village. The only movement in the complex is at the green dome on the south-eastern wall, the tomb to the saint's paternal grandmother, where a number of the shrine's inmates is walking about silently in a circle, ceaselessly and endlessly under the blazing midday sun. They circumambulate the dome of the tomb either clockwise and anti-clockwise, in accordance with a directive that they regard as sacred because it was given to them while they were in trance or during a dream. They walk round the dome on the stony ground without the slightest protection from the sun. All that can be heard is the soft shuffling of their feet and the jingling of the women's glass bangles. They do not even look at the Western woman who is visiting, but simply continue on their circular way, fulfilling their task.

If one descends the some sixty to eighty steps from the dome one encounters an iron grating in front of the paternal grandmother's grave. Hanging from the grating are countless glass bangles that add a splash of colour. The women pilgrims whose ailments have been cured or problems have been solved, or whose wishes for a son, for instance, have been fulfilled, come here, light a candle and hang a bangle on the grating. While I look at the grating and picture to myself the numerous fates which led to this accumulation of tokens of despair and its conquest, a fifteen year-old girl whose ear- and nose-rings show her to be a Rajasthani comes rushing down the steps. She lights a candle and places it on the grating. "What's up with you?" I ask. "*Hajri* ati hai," she answers, "I am entering trance and," she adds, "it's the devil. The devil has entered me." "How do you know?" I ask. "You can tell it's him because he sends you flying to the ground with enormous force when he rises up inside you," she replies, already looking over her shoulder to me as she hurries back up the stairs, as fast as she came.

Dealings with the devil in the early afternoon, I reflect, what a light-footed girl. My culture impressed other notions of footprints on me, and not merely during school lessons in Bavaria, nor simply from the press back then during the most recent case of exorcism in Franconia.[1]

I walk back to the entrance, for the sun is beginning to descend and will soon start to disappear behind the broad plain in a long and glorious sunset. *Goduliwela* as the people here call this timeless hour between day and night — literally the hour in which the cattle are driven back home. We all meet up again at a tea stall. "Tea please", I mutter, "no sugar, just a drop of milk." "Coffee please," says Vikram Nath, "lots of coffee, lots of sugar, lots of milk." And Anil, the owner of the car and our travel companion today, drinks Limca, three bottles one after the other. We are tired now and would like most of all to slump down behind the counter while the others who have come on a pilgrimage emerge from their quarters and assemble.

Because every day at five p.m., one hour before darkness falls, there is a grand evening ceremony with incense, drums and *shehnai*.[2] The incense rises up out of censers which are swung to and fro by the *mujawars* and their assistants. For this they use a small piece of *resina benzoe* or *loban*. The pilgrims purchase it at the entrance and hand it to their *mujawars* to burn in the evening. The *mujawars* also call this evening ceremony the *loban* ceremony or simply *loban* time.

The courtyard of the tomb is already filling up. Lots of brightly dressed women, as well as men, pour through the large archway in which the musicians, who call themselves fakirs, play their drums and shehnai on the first floor. The musicians are father and son, for the positions here at the tomb are inherited. Several years later the father, the shehnai player, died. His son, Ahmad Karim, who was then left on his own to play the large drum, which is the size of a kettle drum, said, "We have no replacements and no descendants who would be willing to do this, so where am I to find someone?" And he added, "My son is only ten, and not even he will want to play here."

The courtyard is full, there is no room left to stand. Hindu women from Rajasthan with silver jewellery and yellowish red saris are standing tightly packed with Muslim women in the long gowns that are normally concealed in public beneath their *burkas*.[3] And the inevitable hordes of adolescent children have also turned up, creating their customary hubbub and disturbances.

Meanwhile the dignitaries of the holy shrine have come and assembled around the main entrance to the tomb. They all wear a dark headdress that resembles a hat without a brim, and a black cloak that reaches to their knees. Underneath this they wear white pyjamas or tight legwear called *churidar*. The seniormost dignitary[4] carries an ornately embellished silver sceptre in his right hand during this ceremony, while in his left he swings a large censer. The courtyard is now so full of people that it is impossible to move of one's own volition; one is pushed, shoved and jostled past the tomb. The dignitaries' prayers can now only be made out by their movements and gestures. The elder swings his sceptre with powerful movements, as do the other dignitaries with their censers. In addition a little holy water from the spring in the tomb is sprinkled over the crowds of the faithful. The saint's power is present wherever there is incense or water.

The initially soft muttering and muffled speech of the crowd grows louder. People start shoving their way from the back in order to get through the entrance. And now the music of the shehnai echoes over to us, permeates the crowd and mingles with the screams that now begin to rend the air and become increasingly shrill. The beats of the drum, which resonate with increasing clarity from the balcony above the gate, speed up the motion of the crowd below, as well as the cries, which are mainly uttered by the women. The air has grown thick with incense, it is scarcely possible to distinguish a single person in the heaving mass. All individuality has been extinguished: everything is one. And everyone is like everyone else.

The time is auspicious, everyone can benefit from the saint's willingness to help. Everyone has established a link with him. The first women start to fall to the ground in trance. Their piercing screams fill the court with their rhythms. Their bodies writhe: "Aah - uee - aaah," they scream, long-short-long, "aah - uee - aah." The veils fall from their bodies, their hair loosens and enters the rhythms of their movements. Eyes closed or their gaze directed inwards, their bodies bump against the walls of the tomb and the small marble walls between the graves of Mira Datar's lesser relatives.

The crowd has grown particularly dense on the terrace around the dome which the inmates of the tomb encircle at the noonday hour. The steps are densely packed. The way up to the terrace is laborious, feet tread on feet rather than the floor. I wind my way up from the bottom step to the top between bodies which can be felt but not seen, and as I at last reach the terrace I spot a woman standing on top of the dome, swinging her hair in a circle before the rosy evening sky. Another woman is trying to make her way to the place on the dome occupied by the first woman, and she too keeps flinging her hair forward with a jerky motion. All the while a dense knot of pilgrims keeps circling round the foot of the dome. Among them is the young girl who had told me that afternoon that she is possessed by the devil. She throws herself forwards towards the dome in a series of daring rolls, and then nimbly repeats them in reverse. Then she walks on all fours and turns her head quickly and wildly in a circle so that her hair flies all around. Her face is anxious when she performs her forward rolls, but triumphant when in the end she finally emerges from her trance. I go over to her, to the corner from which she commences her somersaults. "What is it that's inside you?" I ask. "And where does it come from?" And once again she says: "The devil rises up inside me." "Where from?" I ask. "From my stomach to my head," she replies. "And what happens then?" "It makes me dizzy." "Does it hurt?" I ask. "Yes, it hurts when it rises up," she replies. Then her eyes open wide, she looks straight through me and executes her next somersault towards the dome.

As darkness descends the ecstatic, collective crush begins to ebb. The women pull themselves together, grab hold of their veils, reach out for their companions and straighten their hair and their faces. Only women fall into ecstasy, men adhere to the prayer formulae that the dignitaries recite to them. The congregation slowly disperses from the tomb complex. Occasionally a small group lingers awhile by the walls of the tomb, and the one woman or the other remains convulsed in trance. But the vast majority is now set on visiting the tomb of the maternal uncle outside of the complex. Here the din swells up again, the collective ecstasy surges up one more time, then finally to extinguish. The last cries die away, the congregation returns to its quarters. Night begins, peace is restored. Just the muttering of small groups of pilgrims can still be heard.

We are back inside the car, which is now returning to Ahmedabad. Before Vikram Nath can get absorbed in his betel nut, I say: "Vikram Nath, this is just the right place. This is exactly where I want to work." "I already said that to the *mujawars* when they asked me what we wanted here," he answers, laughing. The red juice from the pan trickles from the corner of his mouth.

We decide to return in September once the monsoon is over. That will allow me time to prepare for the data gathering and to ready myself for all that we have sampled today.

The Tomb and its Order

During the years in which I talked with the possessed women at the Mira Datar Dargah I often held lectures on my impressions and experiences. Sometimes I would let a recording of the *hajri* texts from the tomb run at the same time, or I showed a film or simply slides. On one occasion a member of the Indian diplomatic corps attended a lecture that I gave in Delhi. He was a Muslim from a high caste designated as Ashraf, as opposed to the low-caste *Ajlaf*. He studied the beggars before the gateway, listened to the screams of the women in *hajri*, looked at the pitiful figures snoozing before the door to the grave — all with his strongly traditional, Muslim cast of mind; and scarcely had my last picture disappeared and my last word faded than he vented his indignation at the decline of the culture at the Muslim shrines.

"It is quite inconceivable," he shouted, "that places which were once visited by kings and princes and where they sought to be buried have now succumbed to superstition and the sort of behaviour you would only expect in a whorehouse."

And he continued with the bearing of a schoolmaster: "It was places like these from which Islam was disseminated, this is where the great Islamic mystics taught, and now amulets are being handed out to mentally retarded women," he shouted, then adding quietly, almost sadly: "What a downfall."

My depiction had not met with his pleasure. From his viewpoint he was quite right to feel sad at this "downfall". Muslim shrines, as they are termed in the literature, are an old institution on the Indian sub-continent — one with a strong tradition. When Islam was brought by eighth-century traders to the peninsula of Sind and with that India, it was essential for the Muslims to defend their religion against the Hindus. This was often solved in those days, as indeed now, by martial power. Once however, Islam had come to be the religion of the rulers, and Delhi was ruled by a Sultanate, the mystical Sufi orders rose to became the strongholds of the imported religion. But even before this the orders set up hospices *(khanqah)* and used them for ascetic exercises as well as for service to the community.

The first two Sufi orders were established under the Sultanate of Delhi in the thirteenth century. They were the Chishti and Suhrawardi orders, followed in the fifteenth century by the third, the Qadiri order (Gaborieau, 1986). The fourth great Sufi order, the Naqshbandi order, came in the sixteenth century. The first was founded by Mu'in al-din Chishti (deceased 1233), one of the foremost spiritual leaders of India who established himself, under the escort of the first Islamic troops, in Ajmer in the province of Rajasthan in approximately 1220 A.D., where he founded a *khanqah* in which he was later buried (Currie, 1989). Since the rule of Sultan Akbar (1556–1605), the tomb and the *dargah* of Ajmer are the most important places of Muslim pilgrimage in the sub-continent. The Chishti order is viewed as a purely Indian Sufi order, while the others, such as the second most important, the Suhrawardi order, still has clear connections with its Afghani or Persian origins. The Suhrawardi order was introduced to India at the beginning of the Sultancy of Delhi by three disciples of Shihab al-din 'Umar Suhrawardi (deceased 1234 in Baghdad) (Lawrence, 1978).

The French anthropologist and South Asia expert Gaborieau (1986) writes that, unlike Chishti's followers, the Suhrawardi monks, whose centre was located in Multan (in present-day Pakistan), had close contact with the worldly powers-that-be from the very beginning, and thus received a regular flow of donations for the estates on which they built their monasteries.

Gaborieau (1986) demonstrates in his survey article "*Les Ordres mystiques dans le sous-continent indien*" how various political camps laid claim to the Sufi shrines during their historical development. The Muslim reformers take pains in their publications to represent the dargahs as centres of social regeneration in general, if more importantly of Muslim–Indian society in particular. Gaborieau endeavours to prevent the syncretic elements of the Indian Sufi movement from vanishing into obscurity and to show Indian Sufism as an Indian phenomenon and not simply a Muslim phenomenon.

Syncretism, the intercultural exchange of the elements and contents of various faiths, can also be seen to have occurred between Hindu medicine and the medicine of Islam: the religions and medicines brought to the sub-continent by the immigrants were unable to withstand Hindu influences. Gaborieau (1986) notes that since the fifteenth century Sufi saints have employed yoga techniques to achieve ecstasy. A fine example of the syncretic mingling of the Hindu mystical tradition with Muslim tradition is the mystic and poet Kabir (deceased 1518), who at an early date attempted to resolve the differences between the two religions in his *bhakti* poetry, a form of verse dedicated to the worship of God. This can be seen clearly in the following text, even if it is not intended to be completely straightforward:

Kabir says
that in the hour of death
the Hindu takes the name of Ram
and sings,
while the Muslim
brings Khuda's name
to his lips—
Neither had sung
either of the
names
during their lives

In other places he writes that the Ka'aba of Mecca is now Benares (the Hindu says Kashi and by that means the sacred city of Benares), adding that the Hindu God Ram has now become Rahim, meaning Allah:

The Ka'aba is now Kashi
And Ram is now Rahim
Coarse flour has been ground fine
Come, Kabir, partake of it

Gaborieau writes that the Muslim tombs with their *dargahs* (royal courtyards), where the veneration of the saints is practised, are clearly a vehicle of syncretism and thus never came into the hands of the reformers. This also applies to the tomb described in this book.

The possessed women of the Mira Datar Dargah are, as shall be seen in the following chapters, anything but a vehicle for Islam; they move about on a surface, a stage that is defined by karamat, the saint's power. Their practices are attributed to both popular Hindu and popular Muslim religion. Many similar Muslim saints' tombs are used in India in the way I have described here. Many of them I have visited myself and many more were described to me, but only a very few, of which I would like to mention three, have entered the literature (Basu, 1993; Jeffery, 1979; Rollier, 1982).

While Basu's highly ingenious study centres on the local saint of the Sidis in Gujurat, Bava Gor, and Rollier's analysis of possession and trance at the tomb of Murugmalla focus on a local saint in Bangalore — both with reference to ethno-psychiatric literature — Jeffery presents the shrine of one of the most famous Sufi saints, Nizamuddin, whose *dargah* is located on the edge of New Delhi. Common though to all three shrines is that they act primarily as a centre for local worship. With the exception of Nizamuddin's tomb, which like Ajmer belongs to the "Muslim internationalists", their congregations are ecumenical. Many of the *mujawars* of the Mira Datar Dargah kept repeating to us that formerly the shrine was of national importance and visited by pilgrims from all of the major cities of India. But nowadays, as they all agreed, the majority of visitors came from rural Rajasthan and Gujarat, making it a place of local pilgrimage.

A further characteristic that is often attributed to the Islamic institutions in India is the notion of equality. Yet Islamic society is no less hierarchical and divided into castes than Hindu society. However, the *khanqahs* and *dargahs* were regarded as spiritual centres in which the caste mentality was eliminated in favour of the notion of equality (Gaborieau, 1986). This was replaced though in the Sufi shrines by the unconditional surrender of the pupil (murid) to the spiritual master (*pir* or *murshid*). More particularly this surrender annuls any membership of a specific caste or local group. Gaborieau mentions in his article that the renunciation of caste membership, as practised by the pupils of Kabir or other bhaktas (mystics), or among the Sikhs, is an ancient and constantly recurring practice in Hindu India (1986, p.118).

The Mira Datar Dargah is mentioned on a number of occasions in the nineteenth-century censuses. In the Gazeteer of the Mumbai Presidency of 1899 we find an interesting entry on the shrine's budding fame. It states that the late Gaekwar of the house of the Khanderaos, had become a pious follower of the saint and had a bannister of solid silver built around Mira Datar's tomb to express his gratitude. This silver bannister attracted many pilgrims and believers, thus making the shrine the most famous tomb in all of Gujarat (1899).

The Mira Datar Dargah is something of an exception among Sufi shrines: as we know from the legends, its foundation is based on the saint's martyrdom. The young Mira Datar became a *shahid*, or martyr, during the clashes between the Hindu princes and the sultans. His sainthood is due to his sacrifice, the sacrifice of his young life in the "cause of Islam", and to his "purity", for he went to war unmarried — against the will of his mother who wished to marry him off quickly and somewhat furtively. This is the reason why a mace has been carved at the head of the stone slab on his tomb. This stone sign denotes *shahidana*, martyrdom. Thus Mira Sayed Ali Datar was not a spiritual teacher, not a *murshid* or Sufi saint. Yet all the same the Mira Datar Dargah is assigned to the Sufi shrines, more specifically to those of the Suhrawadi. The reasons for this need some explaining.

When I began my work at the tomb I initially assumed that this was not a Sufi shrine, because it was not founded by a spiritual leader. Confusing in this context was the fact that it is nevertheless mentioned in the governmental census report, the *Gazetteer of Gujurat* (1975), as the grave of a Muslim *pir*, a saint and teacher. The term *pir* is reserved solely for Muslims; Hindus refer to their teachers as gurus. Both mean spiritual teacher. "What sort of shrine is it then?" I asked myself. As did others, such as Imtiaz Ahmad, who wanted to publish my work on it in his book *Ritual and Religion among Muslims in India*, and did so later without my ever answering his question (Ahmad, 1981).

Gaborieau, who is also an ethnographer, recommends a particular means of diagnosis. He writes that in contrast to the Hindu orders, the orthodox Sufi orders are intimately linked with the higher castes (in this case the Ashraf). If a person in these circles senses the slightest likelihood of having descended from a *pir*, best of all one who enjoyed a certain renown, they will live off the religion, which is to say on the takings of the hospice or the tomb. In particular, families in the Pakistani Punjab have attained great power and influence by enlisting such sources. Should they lack the asset of a holy ancestor, they can make their living as a civil servant or such like. "And how can they be recognised," asks Gaborieau as he commences his description of the people. "They can be recognised by their titles, *shah*, *pir* or *khwaja*... or by their surnames, *Chisthi, Suhrawardi, Qadiri, Naqshbandi*..." (Gaborieau, 1986, p.122) or from the graves of their ancestors or such non-specific designations as pirzade, which denotes the descendant of a *Pir*.

Those were enough distinguishing features. The "identikit" picture was perfect. On top of this came the fact that every *mujawar* we talked to at the Mira Datar Dargah gave Suhrawadi (= those who belong to the Suhrawadis) as his surname in our printed questionnaire. Yes, there could be no doubt about it, that's what they were because they tended their sinecures with true devotion. And the fondness they had for the worldly powers-that-be was equally unmistakable.

"When are you going to bring the BBC?" the Suhrawadis at the shrine kept asking me. "Recently a bus full of German tourists arrived here, thanks very much for thinking of us," they said full of praise, even though I certainly was not behind this visit because I had always kept the "address" to myself.

The family genealogies are kept in the office of the *Sajjadanashin*, and are written in Arabic script.

A genealogy begins with Mira Datar's father, Sayed Dosan Miyan, who settled in Unava in 1493, one year after his son's martyrdom, after having already brought his family here in the sixties and with that founded the line of the Suhrawadis in Unava. Mira Datar's dates are given as 1474 to 1492. This genealogy stretches from Mira Datar's father to Muhammadhusen, the *Sajjadanashin* during the period in which I conducted my interviews. A second genealogy consists of a list of the patrilinear ancestors before the saint's time that Dosan Miyan brought with him to Unava, and which only includes the eldest sons. This reads as follows:

"Hazrat Abdul begat Hazrat Hasan Hazrat Hasan begat

Hazrat Amir Hazrat Amir begat Hazrat Imam Hasan Hazrat Imam Hasan begat Hazrat Imam Sainullabadin etc. etc. ..."

Twenty-six generations are listed in this manner. In the first six the title Hazrat is used, and from then on until Mira Datar the names bear the title Sayed. Presumably this title changed after the family emigrated to north India. The title Sayed indicates that the bearer belongs to the upper category of the highest caste, the Ashraf, and in the Indian context it means that the bearer descends from the family of the Prophet. Thus membership of the Sayed stratum is of the foremost social relevance to the families who own the tomb of Nizamuddin (Jeffery, 1979) and the families of Mira Datar. It even ranks higher than their religion (Gaborieau, 1986).

"Sayed girls marry Sayed boys, that is the rule in all Sayed families," as Haji Sayed Miyan, a toothless old *mujawar*, tells me, "... it has always been that way, ever since we came here from Buchara."

However, his next statement makes me feel uncertain: "Because we are from the Chisthi family, we are Naqshbandi, we are Huseni." He names all of the orders, not just those to which family he really belongs. Why did he say that, I ask myself. But when he then says that buses arrive every day with people from Germany, Africa, France and the whole of India, I interpret his words slightly more generally.

What he is saying by this is that we belong to the top ranks of Muslim society and that our shrine is so famous it is known the whole world over. Perhaps he says this because he does not belong to the top ranks of society? Is this a case of deception, of pretending to have a different status, the way many others do? I was slightly worried that I might have made a "wrong diagnosis". But a conversation with Muhammadhusen put my mind at rest.

"They are all Sufi orders, he said, "Chisthi, Suhrawadi, Qadiri, Naqshbandi, and what's more the most important ones. As I told you earlier, and as you wrote in your notes, we call ourselves Suhrawadi. And as for Haji Miyan who told you that," he added after a while, "well he hails from Mahapalli and cannot possibly be a Suhrawadi. The Mahapalli *mujawars* are Hussenis." This made it clear to me that this group, which I will come to discuss in due course, did not belong to the elite as they did.

In addition to this it is also socially important for each of the Suhrawadis of Unava to be able to trace his ancestry back to the saint's father. This is the necessary working basis as it were if one is to draw an income from the shrine. This purely bodily relationship to the sanctity of the place is demonstrated by the family graves. And particularly interesting in this context is their arrangement: very close to Mira Datar is the grave of Dosan Miyan, the father and not least the person who also sent Mira Datar to wage battle against the Hindu king. The saint's community feels that he deserves to be so close. Beside him rests Ilm ul-din, the grandfather, and beside him Bura, the saint's brother's second son, and in between, almost squeezed into place and resting against the holy grave, is the stone slab of his oldest brother Abu Muhammad. The fifth closest grave is of a woman.

What woman, we wondered for a long while, would have been admitted to the strictly male stage of these graves? What importance could she have had? We asked the *mujawars*, who explained the funeral grounds to us. The answer was clear and the only one that could fit the Muslim world picture:

"This is the woman who fed *baba* his milk."

We needed to ask no more. The father's seed determines his ancestry, the milk from (some) woman is his life, his family, so consequently this (nameless) woman is allowed to rest close to him on account of her milk. She is the only woman on this male stage, and her presence is mute. The sixth grave is for the neem twig which the saint was using to clean his teeth when he was called to battle. And finally the seventh grave, set at a respectful distance away in the silver wall that surrounds the men's inner courtyard, contains the King of Mandu who killed the saint, and who likewise was killed by the saint. The tomb symbolises their similarity in death and the antagonism of their causes.

Is there also a grave for Mira Datar's mother, we wondered after hearing this explanation, knowing full well that when the community arranged the graves, it certainly did not "forget" that the mother would rather have had her son married than watch him be killed and turned into a martyr.

"Where is his mother's grave?" I asked Haji Sayed Miyan, Muhammadhusen, and even on one occasion asked Mazar.

"In Mahapalli!" came Mazar's reply, accompanied by a sweeping gesture to the west, in the direction of the ox-carts that were driving off into the sunset in a cloud of dust. So it was just as we thought, his mother's grave had not been allowed inside the shrine, rather it had been placed outside. In all correctness it should be added that it had received its own *dargah*, the *dargah* of Mahapalli which almost everyone visits.

Mahapalli is several miles to the west of the main *dargah*. The pilgrims always include the mother's tomb in their tour. Almost no one leaves the Mira Datar complex without having first paid a visit to the Rastima, as the mother's tomb is called. Rastima's *dargah* is under its own direction. And the Rastima also has its red-letter day once a year: its *urs*, which is celebrated independently of the main shrine, albeit with less pomp. The Rastima *mujawars* wear large, green turbans (in contrast to the small, black caps worn by the administrators of the main *dargah*). The inner courtyard is neat and mostly empty. The funeral chamber of the saint's mother, the Rastima, is painted turquoise green. Wooden doors lead inside. The grave may not be visited by male pilgrims, for a female saint is resting there. But I should hasten to add that the women have not succeeded in capturing it as their own stage, because no one apart from the *mujawars* may enter. Bright lengths of thread have been wound round the tomb railings. There are places inside the inner courtyard where small miracles occur. There is an opening in one of the walls, for instance, into which the pilgrims can call and then hear their voice echo repeatedly from out of the walls. The atmosphere at Rastima's *dargah* is different to that of the main *dargah*. It is easier, more playful.

Haji Sayed Miyan tells me how Rastima's court came into being, and from where her *dargah* received its name:

"It was during the time of the Mughal rule that Mira Sayed

Ali Shihad Datar made his sacrifice. In those days it was the custom for the king to give a present or a girl of his own choice to those who made great sacrifices or won a battle or distinguished themselves in some other way. After Mira Datar had made his sacrifice the king wished to reward him, so he sent him a girl. He sent him his Mahapalli, his special companion. Her name was Darbibi. He sent her escorted by numerous servants. And they came here. The king gave them land and property. They received the land during the reign of King Ahmad Shah. And they built on the land and called it Mahapalli after Darbibi. Mira Datar's mother, Rastima, who no longer wished to remain in Unava, is buried in Mahapalli."

"Shortly after, Mira Sayed Shihad Ali Datar was brought here to Unava. He was buried here because he told his father to do so in a dream: `Take me to Unava, and make a grave for me under the neem tree. All who come to my grave will have their wishes granted and their illnesses cured.'

"And according to the legend, in a second dream he made a further request to his father: 'And bury the head of King Mahendi, whom I slew, in the same temple.'"

Haji Sayed Miyan concluded his story by adding: "The neem tree has remained green to this day." Women who want a child but have not yet given birth can conceive if they take a leaf from the tree.

The tracks of the women in the myth of Mira Datar lead to Mahapalli. They are not part of the official myth at the tomb, the myth that is told by men — and only by men. The bit of "official" myth that is allowed the women at the Mira Datar complex has been removed and placed elsewhere. It begins with the sacrifice of the beautiful young Darbibi to the dead Mira Datar. Her court contains the grave of mother Rastima, who did not wish to sacrifice her son for either a war or a religion. This court of the clever women has no "history," and if it had its story would in any case have become another. But the court of Mahapalli gives an idea of this history, for it is bright and cheery. Perhaps this is the picture that people have of women in Islam: a woman who wishes to serve the family, their politics and help its continued existence must be licked into shape, circumcised and veiled. Anyone who fails to comply will have to live "outside". But it can by all means be beautiful and stimulating out there, perhaps even nicer than inside. Every pilgrim goes to Rastima once in order to receive her blessing as well.

"We're going to Mahapalli," Tajinder's mother called to me before their departure. Her words had a ring of gaiety about them. "Have you already been to Rastima?" we were often asked. It sounds like a lovely prospect, like a trip into the country.

So what was at the back of Muhammadhusen's remark about the *mujawars* at Mahapalli? As we arrived in Unava and began our interviews, it was explained to us at some point that the administrators of Mahapalli did not have a lot to do with them. I asked straight out: "Would any of you marry their daughters?" This was met by an incensed silence, followed by a faint smile and finally:

"No, never, you see they came here as servants. The king in fact gave the land to us and we paid them for their services, for the ceremonies, etc. ... so how could we marry their women?"

But if one goes to Mahapalli and talks with the *mujawars* there — there are almost thirty of them in all — about the order of their shrine, they will say that they are descended from Mira Datar's oldest brother, Abu Muhammad. And when, during the second year of our research, we handed out questionnaires to each of the *mujawars* who works with the pilgrims, the Mahapalli *mujawars* quite truthfully entered their names as Husseni and not Suhrawadi. So they did belong to a different group. But they were unable to talk about it.

Rastima is also economically independent of the main shrine. The system is however the same. There is also a *golakh* here, a donation box for the shrine's income, and the *mujawars* also receive direct incomes from their personal clients. The difference lies solely in the fact that economic matters are conducted far less openly here than among the Suhrawadis. The *mujawars* of Unava told us that Rastima was built a century ago and that the shrine is now one hundred years old.

When a pilgrim enters the courtyard here and turns to a *mujawar*, the latter will also tie a red cord round the pilgrim's wrist the way his colleagues do at the main shrine, and, taking the other end, tie it to one of the silver columns by Rastima's grave so that she will "take on" the case. The pilgrim then recites the following prayer:

> Oh Rastima, I am tethering myself
> in your court by a ribbon
> link me with the grace that you
> bestow upon me, drive the
> bhut, the balla, the churäl and the
> *dakin* and the evil *jinn* at home
> away from me,
> take these spirits, this sickness, away
> make everything good
> by your mercy, Rastima...

Although the client may then undergo her *hajri* procedure in the main shrine, she feels bound to Rastima. Without doubt the male saint is regarded as the more powerful. But there are always a few pilgrims who tether themselves here. Everything at Rastima's court is gentler, even the punishments — compared with those we observed in Mira Datar's court. There are just two: either one plunges into the water tank or one sits in the sewage water. And I have never seen anyone having to perform either of them at Rastima's court. Nobody was lying face down in the gully, as can often be seen at the main shrine. Women sauntered through the courtyard, would also sometimes go into a trance, and then withdrew to a shady corner to rest. The water tank in Rastima's court has a smaller, separate basin set inside the main one. The latter is employed for the customary ablutions performed in Islamic rites, the smaller basin for battles when exorcising demons.

"It's imperative," explains Jamiat Miyan, one of the oldest *mujawars* at Rastima's tomb, "because the demons make the water so incredibly filthy that we could no longer expect anyone to use it for their ablutions before their prayers."

Close to Mahapalli is Kacheria, the location of the saint's

lawcourt. It catches the eye as a result of its immense silver chair upholstered with red velvet. Two smaller chairs have been set to the left and the right of the large silver chair. The place is looked after by the Mahapalli *mujawars*. They look after the shrine and in the evening collect the banknotes that are placed before the sacred chair. The pilgrims place their cases before the court chair in the form of small handwritten notes. The whole shrine consists of just one small building before which the women lie in *hajri* or kneel in prayer. Kacheria's silver chair was donated some thirty years ago by a rich Parsi who was healed at the Mira Datar complex.

"He gave us twenty thousand rupees," one of the *mujawars* says with satisfaction, "twenty thousand rupees for the silver chair."

The women say, "Baba comes by night and casts judgement and fulfils the pilgrims' wishes. If you come here during the night and observe the chair from the distance, you can see baba sitting there and attending to his court work." *Baba* is a tender expression for the childlike saint. When the saint was a child— "for he was a saint from birth," as legend has it — he held court beneath the neem tree. On becoming a martyr he continued to hold court in invisible form. Some people see him in their dreams examining the petitions cases that the visitors place before the chair.

"Do you work with dreams?" we asked the Mahapalli *mujawars* in order to discover whether they have a different healing tradition to that of the main shrine.

"Yes, of course we work with dreams! How else are we find out when the cure has been completed? This always reveals itself in dreams. When they dream that they are tying up their bed-rolls or sitting on a train or returning to their families, we know that we can give them the recommendation *(hukm)* to set off home," says Jamiat Miyan as he explains his duties to us in his office.

"Can you also interpret complicated dreams?" we ask. "If the dream is too complicated we ask baba to send us a new one that is easier to interpret," Jamiat Miyan replies.

"I, too, had a dream that left a deep impression on me

and kept me thinking," Jamiat Miyan says, and he divulges his dream to Vikram Nath and myself:

"Mira Datar was holding court. Fifty-two pious followers had come and were seated in a circle at the saint's feet. I was sitting right at the end in a corner. Cold drinks were served up in wonderful cups on magnificent trays. Sorbets in every imaginable colour were being offered. The cups were passed round the group of people at the feet of the saint in a circle, but I was the last and there was never enough for me as well. I threw the empty cup away in anger, got up and left."

"I interpreted the dream for myself," he continued, "I am out of luck, I failed to receive Mira Datar's grace. I was a young, angry man in those days, but now I have grown calmer."

This dream means more, though. Jamiat Miyan belongs to the "second-class" *mujawars*, to those from Mahapalli who do not come from a Sufi order and may even have descended from servants. Might not this private dream have summed up the collective problem of the Mahalapalli *mujawars*?

In Chapter V, I will often come to speak of Dadima's dome at the tomb which the pilgrims walk round in a circle, and on which women stand during *hajri*, and which also plays a part in the "punishments" when it is encircled in a particular manner. Dadima's grave is situated on the south-east corner of the outer wall of the main courtyard. The grave is a good fifty steps below the surface of the earth, and the dome is two storeys above. It has been painted green but it is well-worn from the never-ending circumambulations round the grave. Dadi means father's mother in Hindi and Urdu, so Dadima's grave is that of Mira Datar's paternal grandmother. Once again we have here a woman's grave that has been placed in a prominent position, but virtually outside of the main complex. Nothing in the legends I heard said anything about the paternal grandmother. Yet the grave is important. It is no less a part of the cult than the main grave. The women allow many of their manifestations to occur before Dadima or on the dome. And it also has a certain uniqueness, as has already been alluded to: women like to offer glass bangles to Dadima by attaching them to the grating before the grave. Such offerings are also made though to (Hindu) mother goddesses over the whole of India. Consequently the grating before Dadima's grave is decorated in the manner of a Hindu goddess.

Dadima has power because she gives strong *hukms* (advice). A woman who each day held her head in the sewage water for hours on end answered our disconcerted questions by saying: "That is Dadima's *hukm*." And another woman who received the hukm from Dadima to return home, but did not obey, soon became confused and then *pagal* or crazy. She had to be fetched by her relatives and taken home, where she was quickly restored.

The pilgrims walk from one grave to the next on the *hukm* of one of the saints. The inner geography of pilgrimage at the tomb is a product of dream-and trance-texts. They read their dreams together with the *mujawars* and then determine their round of prayers for that day or week. The route through the grave complex is determined by the subconscious. "Why are you here in Mamasahib's tomb," we often asked, "or at Rastima's tomb?" And the answer was always: "*Hukm*. It was the *hukm* of baba or Dadima or Mamasahib".

Dadima and Rastima, the mothers, hold the outposts. They are powerful authorities in the cult at the Mira Datar tomb. They are part of the women's stage, but they are hardly mentioned in the legends related by the men.

On the road to the north, half a mile from the Mira Datar Dargah, is the tomb of Rastima's brother, Hazrat Hamza. His grave bears the word for maternal uncle: *Mamasahib*. It is primarily visited during the evening incense ceremony, by all of the pilgrims, and gets so full that one can no longer find the stone floor beneath one's feet. The tomb of *Mamasahib*, or Mamusahib as it is generally called, is also a permanent part of the ritual proceedings. It is the smallest of the tombs, but it has its own roofed courtyard which surrounds the grave. The takings from the Mamasahib tomb and the Dadima tomb are auctioned off once a year among the *mujawars*. Whoever makes the highest bid receives the bonus, the *mujawar*-ship, and with that he gets the takings from the pilgrims who tie their threads to the pillars of the tomb. Five per cent of this must be handed over though to the government's "Reservation Fund".

The officiating *mujawars* are responsible for the running of the rituals. Each week one of them assumes the overall responsibility for the entire Mira Datar complex. This duty is shared amongst nine families. The *mujawar* in charge goes to the *dargah* at four a.m. The first day of this duty is always a Friday, the holy day. After washing his hands and feet he enters the burial chamber. He removes the faded flowers, takes off the *gilaf*, the shroud, and replaces it with a fresh one. Then he places fresh flowers on the grave and lights the censers. After he has completed his work on Mira Datar's grave he goes and tends the other graves in the courtyard. He must also ensure that small cloth horses are made from the shroud from the grave, which are then swung "125 times" in a circle above the pilgrim's head during the admission ceremony and represent Mira Datar's army.

During the grand incense ceremony in the evening, he goes up to the tomb bearing a silver sceptre whose tip is adorned with the star and moon of Islam, and which is enfolded in a green banner. He speaks the *fatiha*, the first sura of the Koran, and after the ceremony each of the *mujawars* come out and blesses "his" pilgrims. The fakirs carry their censers, and the younger *mujawars* scatter rose petals from the grave over the crowd. Then the *mujawars* sit down with their pilgrims or patients, recite the *saluk* prayer and tie a red thread around the pilgrim's wrist and the saint's silver pillar:

> Oh Datar Baba,
> Oh father the giver of all,
> Look down upon me
> Among the circle of believers
> As I tie the red thread
> Here against them all, the
> *Bhut, palit, churäl, jinnat, japadi*
> *meladi, sikatori* and *vir*
> Because someone from my family
> Gave me of the magic in my food and drink,

Someone from my family, someone close to me
Someone who is a stranger.
Oh Datar Baba with your power
Oh Dadima with your power
Oh Rastima with your power
Oh Mamusahib with your power
Bring him forth
Within three days,
Burn him, turn him to cinders,
Purify my body
And drive away
All of my suffering
For ever.

This prayer is repeated a number of times by the pilgrim. Here at the main shrine all of the "secondary" saints are included as well, a clever step which shows where the real headquarters are.

At each ceremony the *mujawars* send out the horses of the saint's army. These cloth horses are sent five times five times five, i.e one hundred and twenty-five times round the pilgrim's head because, as legend has it, the army consisted of 125,000 warriors. With that the pilgrim is placed in contact with Mira Datar. In addition they bless each of the pilgrims by delivering them a couple of blows with a bunch of peacock feathers. The peacock is often seen as a symbol of rejuvenation, of reincarnation and immortality, as well as of love. The peacock is also linked symbolically with the sun and the tree. No doubt the peacock feathers are associated here with release from spirit possession. They indicate a new beginning, a birth into a new life.

Apart from the *mujawars*, the "ruling administrative class", there are three other groups that belong to the shrine. The first consists of the fakirs. They wake the officiating *mujawar* early in the morning, accompany him during his work inside the shrine, fill the oil lamps and censers, and dry the rose petals that are removed from the slab over the grave. They also fetch the left-over oil from the lamps on the following day, which the *mujawars* use later the same day to massage the patients' heads and legs. Another fakir group, the *rawalia*, plays the drums and shehnai, a kind of oboe, during the incense ceremony. And the *bhangis*, the "sweepers" as they are generally referred to and who can always be seen cleaning the floors, constitute the third group which unceasingly tends to specific tasks at the shrine.

When a pilgrim or patient donates his own weight in goods, such as rice, sugar or blossoms, etc., this is shared among the three groups. "Let's take one rupee fifty for example," Muhammadhusen explains to us. "The fakirs receive 25 paise, the *bhangis* 25, the *mujawars* 35 and the *dargah* 65... or if it is goods, then the fakirs receive half a kilo, the *bhangis* half a kilo, the *mujawars* half a kilo and the *dargah* one kilo."

Some of the pilgrims take a brick with them when they leave. They first carry it round the holy grave with them, then they have it blessed by the *mujawars* and perhaps leave it for a few nights at the saint's tomb so that it will become empowered with *karamat*, healing energy. Then when they are back home they look for a suitable place to build a model of the grave for the saint using this brick. A "grave" of this kind is termed a *chilla* or memorial shrine. *Chilla* is also the name of the forty-day retreat for meditation performed by the Sufis. In Chapter III there is a description of our visit to a *chilla* in Mumbai. There is a Mira Datar-*chilla* network across northwest India. I have visited the *chillas* in Mumbai and Pune, and although we learned of a number of others in Maharashtra and Madhya Pradesh during our work at the tomb. There are certainly many more than just those we heard about. In this way a Mira Datar pilgrimage geography has come into existence. Many of the pilgrims we came to know and spoke with told us that they had first heard about Unava, the main centre, at a local commemorative shrine, and had first spent many days in the *chilla* in order to be healed. However, they had then been told that they should go to the main shrine and would receive help there.

Gaborieau writes in his study on Sufi shrines in India: "Nothing has remained of the great hospices of the middle ages (1986, p.121), ... but the orders live on, ... and are most alive in the worship of local saints, and less so as a means of pursuing a mystical way of life ... (p.128)."

But nowhere in the literature on the Muslim shrines and tombs can one read about the artful women who make their voices heard here. Or how they transformed themselves in the courtyards surrounding the tombs by means of their dreams, texts and dramas. These must remain sub- or anti-texts, otherwise they would be mere legends and no longer alive. The fact that they are still alive will be shown in the next three chapters.

NOTES

1. During the seventies a case of reputed demonic exorcism close to Würzburg, Germany, caught the attention of the press; the victim, a student named Anneliese Michel, was tortured to death by "her" priest.
2. *Shehnai* is a kind of oboe.
3. A *burka* is the black overgarment worn by Muslim women in Indian and the near East. In Iran it is called *chador*. The atmosphere at the tomb demands a process of opening up to the outside. The segregation from the public sphere, as well as the wearing of a veil or *burka*, is eliminated. The women may even wear their hair loose, which is also unavoidable during trance. Thus women have extended here their normal, domestic space.
4. The leading dignitaries of the centre number themselves among the descendants of the saint's brother and are thus blood relatives. With this they legitimate their positions and their role in the administration of the tomb. They are termed *sajjadanashin*.

Chapter 5

The Women's Stage

Cult and Cure at the Mira Datar Dargah I

Dramatis Personae I

We have returned. We have taken two rooms in the Vijay Guest House, a small, simple hotel in Mehsana, for twenty rupees a night. That was $ 2.50 at the time.

We take the bus each day to Unava and the tomb. Judging by the arsenal of research equipment we are carrying with us, we could be driving off to war: cameras and film, tape recorders and cassettes, personal questionnaires for the pilgrims and the patients, personal questionnaires for the *mujawars*. But that is not all: Vikram Nath, who will conduct the interviews with the *mujawars*, has advised me to take on an assistant who will transcribe the taped conversations on site, in the hotel room. We have found her. Her name is Angana and she has a master's degree in German from the University of Delhi. She did the transcriptions and translated them from Hindi into English, a task that required unflagging stamina and dedication. For this she earned the double of a teacher's wages, which she certainly can use, for she will shortly be marrying. Later on we received sporadic visits from a German therapist who was being trained as a psychoanalyst, and a German psychiatrist. I shall call them Dr. Hans and Dr. Irmgard, just as the *mujawars* did. I asked them both to help me at short notice should any questions arise relating to psychiatric matters. Both of them were able to do so during various stages of my study of the Mira Datar tomb, and without asking for remuneration. Perhaps the experience was reward enough. We worked during these phases from the early morning to midnight; in the evening we would check and compare our notes from that day and go through the transcriptions with Angana.

These working evenings always began though with an incredibly good Punjabi meal at a Sardarji's[1] next to our hotel, where the truck drivers went. Sardarji often helped us when we had questions about the names of places of pilgrimage or the like. He became a permanent fixture in our daily routine.

On a number of occasions we were visited by female students who were writing their theses on allied subjects for their anthropology degrees. One of them, whom we can call Wanda, remained longer.

Dramatis Personae II

The following sections will deal with the people who worked at the tomb or who stayed there in order to be cured. These people saw and viewed us — the group described above — as a team. Our arrival meant a confrontation for them which was not to remain without its effect, for it churned them up and triggered reactions that left us speechless and produced real changes in us. The dramatis personae II are the "subject" of the following chapter, just as we were their "subject" while we were working there and made their actions and life histories our "subject". The data that they gave us unreservedly, the real insights into their lives, led us to grasp the social complexity in which they lived.

My questions about this and my curiosity as to how possession and trance are dealt with on an everyday level was turned into "data" by the meeting of Groups I and II and their activities during these encounters — data which led me to understand the question and ultimately to this book. The people in Group II will each be introduced when they make their first entrance.

The Body, its Demon and the Hair: the Balla

As we arrived one morning at the office of

Muhammadhusen, the highest dignitary, we were greeted with a warm welcome. He was sitting on a cushion in front of a mountain of files in which he was writing notes. This was his list of "customers," the addresses of the pilgrims who must be reminded of the positive powers of the sacred tomb. In this way Muhammadhusen kept a tally of his congregation as well as his finances. His son Mazar, a tall, attractive man, had already spotted us at the bus stop and called out that he had a "case" for us. Muhammadhusen used the same expression. "It's a good day today," he said, "a cure has been achieved after a long and demanding period of suffering for the whole family." And while he was still speaking, he rose slowly from his cushion and led us out to the courtyard before the tomb.

We are greeted by the sight of a small group of seated people. An elderly but very powerful woman with grey hair is singing and accompanying herself on the cymbals. Faced towards the tomb, she is singing a song of praise or *bhajan* to the saint. From time to time she raises her arms and underscores her praises to the saint with gestures. Sitting in front of her is a young woman with her back to the grave. Her hair is very curious. It is uncombed and completely dishevelled, such that her face, which is gazing almost apathetically into the distance, is framed by a whole series of knots of tangled hair. Her eyes are empty and unfocussed. "That's her brother," Muhammadhusen says, pointing to the young man sitting beside her. We go and join the group, and others come and join us. A woman behind me whispers: "They're going to cut off her hair because the *balla*[2] is sitting in it." "The *balla* has fallen in love with Tajinder's hair," whispers another woman. "But Tajinder never allowed the *balla* to let down her long, beautiful hair," the first woman adds. I look over questioningly to Muhammadhusen. Meanwhile Mazar, Muhammadhusen's son, has come up to us and says: "While Tajinder was at home in Vilaspur she wanted to go to a festival, which is what she did. But while she was there the *balla* fell in love with her hair. She came here and remained for forty days. During her trance the *jinn*[3] asked for a little more time and said that he would then leave her. Since the *jinn* had in any case announced his intention to depart from the girl, the *mujawars* advised her to make her preparations for her home journey. But while she was away they continued sending out the saint's horse army for her,[4] for forty whole days," Mazar continued. "Well, the girl felt the presence of the spirit two or three times while she was back home in Vilaspur, which is to say she experienced *hajri*." The family sent written reports of what she said during her episodes to Muhammadhusen and his son Mazar. They wrote down what they had heard from Tajinder's lips during *hajri*, that the spirit that had brought about this evil had made its home in her hair. Their letter was received by the *mujawar* who was looking after her, and he wrote back immediately with the recommendation *(hukm)* that her hair should be shorn off completely in front of the saint's tomb, as soon as was humanly possible. I ask: "Why has the girl so many knots and tangles in her hair?" "The *napakjinnat*," says Muhammadhusen, which here means roughly the adverse spirits or quite simply evil, "which has fallen in love with Tajinder's hair has forbidden her to comb it. So it is full of lice and dandruff and knots and tangles." Put in this way, it sounds as though she is about to be given a set of measures for her personal hygiene.[5]

But I don't trust her. "How did the *balla* actually come to be in her hair?" Mazar goes back to the very beginning in order to give a full explanation of his viewpoint.

"*Ballas*, or we also say *bhuts*, are spirits that roam around freely and attempt to enter the body of living human beings. They can only achieve this if their victims are careless."

"What do you mean by careless?" I ask.

"Well, women must take especial care," he says, dropping his voice slightly, "about where they go to and what they do there."

"What exactly?" I ask.

"For instance, it is essential that a woman never relieves herself on her own at a crossroad."

The Hindi expression that he uses is quite direct and leaves no room for mistakes.

"But if they do relieve themselves there a *balla* can enter them. You see, women are *napak*[6] when they have their period.

And the *ballas* are simply waiting for that. They will immediately possess a woman if she is not extremely cautious in what she does. So women should never be more than forty paces away from a horse or an ox, because spirits never stay in the proximity of these animals. But they should also not sit facing the direction in which the spirits have gone; one can always recognise this from their footprints. The footprints of spirits always point in the reverse direction. Our women never urinate at a place that is unsafe. And the men always remove the drops of urine afterwards with water. That is purifying and keeps the *bhut* away."

His explanations impress me, they seem to hit the mark. Apart from which I now recall that whenever we travelled in the evening or passed through villages at dusk, we had always seen the women squatting in rows along the roadside in order to relieve themselves collectively and thus under control.

"All of the women here who go into trance, who have problems and are feeling bad, have a *balla* in them. It is simply because they have not protected themselves," says Mazar, concluding his explanation.

While we were listening to Mazar relate the story of Tajinder from Vilaspur, the *nai*[7] or village barber arrived. The barber, a scrawny man dressed in white and with long, very thin fingers, opens his hair-dresser's bag and, without saying a word, sets to work on Tajinder's hair. She, the possessed victim of a spirit that nobody has identified, remains silently seated while the *nai* cuts off her hair in bunches and hands them to Tajinder's mother, who places them in a tin. The tin is from a common make of margarine, and the brand name, "Dalda," can still be seen on it. Once Tajinder's hair has been completely shorn, her mother continues the song of praise that had been interrupted by the operation. The *nai* packs his utensils into his bag and leaves. The family gets up and departs to the shops. The young woman covers her shaven head provisionally with her *dupatta*, her cloth veil. Angana and I follow her as she goes outside and takes a seat at one of the tea stalls outside the tomb with her brother and mother.

"How do you feel now without your hair?" we ask her,

still struggling with our own feelings about this "amputation".

"What does it really matter, my hair will grow again," she replies.

"My God, it'll take ages," Angana exclaims, "you had such long hair!" And I was unclear in my mind whether Tajinder's reply had been made in the spirit of resignation, or was caused by indifference and lethargy.

In order to keep tabs on the developments, Angana and I take up quarters next to Tajinder's family. We move in that evening with a water pot, a mat to sit on and the key. We have taken residence in an old, dilapidated town house that belongs to Muhammadhusen. He has rented us one of the rooms for 40 rupees a month.

The next morning as we return from the tea stall we find Tajinder's mother, who we can call Bolabai,[8] in front of her door washing the breakfast dishes. We sit down beside her, but we do not have to ask any questions because she is happy to have someone who will listen to the story of Tajinder and herself. Yet despite this I reflect that the methods we use to gather our "data" are pretty sophisticated.

Tajinder is the sufferer in this family. She takes little part in the general chores, such as running the household, making plans, cooking and such like. She can just about manage to take care of herself. She leaves the problems of attending to her illness to the others. She only talks about inconsequential matters, about what one should do, and perhaps a little about one could do. One could finish one's vocational training, or one could visit relatives. She only says things like that, nothing else. She has annexed a space which makes her noncommital, which protects and which nobody can penetrate.

"The last time we came," says Bolabai, "the *mujawars* gave Tajinder a *ta'widh*.[9] We took it back home with us, where she removed the *ta'widh* and hid it somewhere. We couldn't find it anywhere. Afterwards she didn't have a period for five months. So then we returned here. She was given a new amulet. Her period returned. Then we all drove back home again. And once again she hid the amulet, and her period stopped. She hasn't had one since then. Tomorrow the *mujawars* are going to give her a new amulet. I'll make sure that this time it doesn't disappear again. I've had enough of all this business."

And after a pause she continued: "Tajinder's sickness began when she was sixteen. She came back one day from school and was crying. She didn't sleep any more at night, she simply cried and screamed. Her situation continued to get worse. By the end it got to the point that she went wherever she happened to be and didn't use the toilet any more. For years we had to eat out because our house had turned into a terrible state."

That evening as we discuss the history of Tajinder's illness with Irmtraud, the doctor, she gives us her impressions of the girl. She suspects that she has a slight hormonal dysfunction which she refers to as Basedow's disease. Naturally she can't say for sure because she lacks any data for a proper interpretation. Apart from which she terms her lack of menstruation "psychosomatic amenorrhoea". This medical explanation is a good supplement to the explanation we have arrived at from cultural science.

Young women in this society go through a traumatic and highly stressful phase during precisely the age which marked the onset of Tajinder's illness. It is an epoch in life in which the parents look for a suitable match for their children. From roughly her fifteenth year on a young woman witnesses the way that envoys are sent from other families, speak with their parents, size her up with their eyes and gather information about her. This procedure, which ends with her being transplanted into an utterly foreign household, is doubtless unbearable for some. The young woman finds herself completely defenceless and unable to see any way out. Numerous young women have told me and others much the same thing. Angara had also suffered from this and solved the dilemma by taking a step forward: she accepted the second "offer" but not without first scrutinising her prospective in-laws thoroughly. Tajinder reacted in her own way. A way which is very common here at the tomb and indeed forms a distinct category: women of marrying age find that they are possessed by a *balla* which can destroy the intended order in every imaginable way.

Tajinder cultivated two forms of possession. The first is what made her ill and altered her body: her possible Basedow disease and her amenorrhoea. The latter moreover is a "political" symptom: if Tajinder does not have a period, her family is faced with unbearable uncertainty. Is she pregnant, sick, or possessed by a *balla*? All three possibilities upset the order of the family and turn everything upside down.

The second form of possession, the regularly occurring trance which underlines the first form, restores order inasmuch as it provides the family members with reports on what is happening. They are full of relief when they hear the words that Tajinder's lips utter at the tomb while in trance:

"I have come so that you will leave me. I implore you to leave me!" And they accept the answer given by the *balla*: "I shall leave you, but I still like it in your hair!"

As we know, this led directly to the act of cutting off her hair which documented Tajinder's final release from the *balla* and designated her as "healed".

The hair is both the symbol and the seat of sexual energy. The way a woman does her hair shows her social position: unmarried girls wear two plaits, married women just one. In her study *Medusa's Hair*, Obeyesekere defines a religious virtuoso by her hairdo (Obeyesekere, 1981). She is a woman who has renounced her former status in order to live and work as an ascetic. For this reason she no longer combed her hair and it had become matted. With that her hair had returned to being a part of nature. A woman's hair shows her social location and status. She defines herself by her hair. The chaste and virtuous woman ties her hair up; the available woman wears it down and keeps it glossy; widows and nuns bid farewell to their hair and have it shorn off completely; the possessed woman tosses her hair about while in trance. Draupadi in the great Hindu epic the *Mahabharata* wears her hair loose and smeared with blood as long as her marital status remains unresolved. And only once her love life has been placed in a socially acceptable order does she put her hair back in the order that everyone desires (Hiltbeitel, 1981). "Tajinder's hair reached to her feet," her brother said to Vikram Nath, "she had really beautiful long hair."

Tajinder will not let anybody comb her hair. She refuses to be massaged with the oil blessed by Mira Datar at his tomb. Her sexual energy is not available, cannot be domesticated, not in the sense of a marital contract. We can read this from her hair. And her symptoms of possession, such as her amenorrhoea, tell the same because a person's body will not lie when the social person is caught in a conflict. The symptoms tell us that she is not ready, not now at least, to change over to the role of a woman. Her body is pleading for a postponement. And this is also what she says in trance, what her *balla* says from her: "I shall leave you, but I still like it in your hair."

Bolabai, her mother, is neither willing nor able to deliberate over the signals that Tajinder is giving. She will not tolerate any postponement, and decides to destroy every sign of obstruction. Her daughter's hair is removed and buried at an unknown spot. She will not tell her daughter where, even if she asks.

"How can I tell her?" she asks to us imploringly, "It's really the *balla* that wants to know where her hair is, and," she continues, "do you know what she said to me when we first came here and attended the *loban* ceremony?"

"No, what did she say?"

"She screamed 'you old witch' at me and 'what are you going to do with me? Are you trying to kill me, what's the meaning of all this? You want to kill me!'"

As Angana muttered "O how awful!" Bolabai continued with: "That was naturally just the *balla* speaking in her." And Angara replied obediently: "Yes, that could only have been the *balla*."

But no one said: "A daughter would never say such a thing."

Yet Bolabai felt sufficiently sure of herself to be able to act. The resistance had to be removed. The hair had to be shorn off. And she acted quite correctly in accordance with "official" the way women are talked about. After all, everyone wanted the *balla* to leave the girl.

But at the same time, by having her daughter's head shorn she had assigned her to a place among the widows, the nuns and the sexless women who have to beg for their food.

Vikram Nath, who had not witnessed the girl having her hair cut off, asked Bolabai: "What did Tajinder look like while her hair was being cut off?"

"Oh," she answered, "her face turned a deep, deep red, as if too much heat was rising up to her head, that's how red her face was."

Bolabai, which means the chatterbox, and this is naturally not her real name, is pointing to the heat in Tajinder's face while her hair was being shorn. With that she is saying that her daughter is uncontrollable. I had watched while Tajinder's hair was being cut off. Her face wasn't the slightest bit red. Bolabai is using the metaphor "heat" to indicate uncontrollable.

Previously she had told me that at the beginning of her illness, Tajinder had returned from school with a fever, and, thinking that the heat of the fever had risen to her head, had given her daughter plenty to drink. But the cool drinks that she gave her had been to no avail. "How was I to know that it was a *balla* in her head?" she asks.[10]

The mother, the daughter and the other members of the family talked with one another about the *balla* in Tajinder's head as if it was a part of them, a part that had to be got rid of because it acted unpredictably. So they set off. They went five times to Tajuddin Baba's tomb in Nagpur. But it was of no help. Then three times to the Baba Badbagsingh Sodi temple in the Punjab, but Tajinder threw the amulets aside.

"Didn't you ever ask a doctor what was wrong with her?" one of us asks in astonishment.

"Of course, we went to a doctor when the heat rose to her head at the beginning of the illness, but she threw all the medicines away immediately after," answers Bolabai.

"But the *balla* was also silent at that time," she continues, "Tajinder could do her apprenticeship as a tailor and we all had peace for a while. Then when the *balla* made itself felt again we heard about a *chilla*,[11] which we then visited, as well as the name Mira Datar and this place here."

"Already on our second visit I dreamt about two nights in a row about a young man who came to my bed and said: 'Don't worry, your daughter will be fine again. The *balla* will leave her. It will all just have to run its course.' That's what I dreamt," Bolabai tells us. And Vikram Nath asks, almost in excitement: "What did the young man look like?"

"It was a sixteen year-old boy with an impressive face. It was the sixteen year-old Mira Datar who appeared to me," she replies. "And as he said, she got better because," she continues, "in front of Tajuddin Baba's tomb the *balla* called out in Tajinder's trance: 'Can you hear me? Can you see me? You've been looking for me, search, search for me here, there!' It sounded as if he wanted to entice her back and forth across the whole country."

And we are reminded of what she had called out in her trance here, as Bolabai uttered the words: "So when we arrived here and Tajinder was in *hajri* the *balla* called from her: `I have come in order to get rid of you!' Isn't that right?" she asks, looking at her son, before adding: "We have seen signs of improvement and a cure since we came here and attached the red ribbon to the tomb and to her wrist. Today she even allowed her head to be massaged for the first time with the holy oil."

And Muhammadhusen, the dignitary, even dreamt that the ribbon for her discharge, the *chalu chillai*, could now be tied round her wrist and that she could leave here under the protection of the horses. And Bolabai had also had a dream in which she saw herself riding in a train with her family.

And what does Tajinder say? She says a lot, about all sorts of things, such as film stars, kings and queens and her relatives, but only third persons. She only says one thing about herself: Tajinder gives me some information which tallies with what the young woman from Rajasthan said whom I met the day I arrived. Both say independently of one another: "You can feel the heat in your body, there's a strange feeling inside you which rises up and can even reach your head, and then you no longer know what you're doing."

The young woman from Rajasthan called "it" the devil. Tajinder (and her family) called "it" the *balla,* the evil spirit. The thing that rises up is treated by the person concerned and their social surroundings as if it were some disturbing factor. But let us take a closer look at it.

Tajinder warded off all the things she was given to make "it" disappear. She either hid them or she threw them away. Perhaps she wanted "it" to happen?

"Hajri ati hai" — "a presence rises up in me" — as the young women say here at the tomb. What kind of presence? What do the women do with it? What do they use it for?

Tajinder's story is viewed as finished. The family is preparing to return home after visiting all the tombs of the saint's relatives one last time. It is five kilometres to Rastima, Mira Datar's mother. They will have to hire a motor rickshaw. Oil will have to be bought, as well as *loban,* and Bolabai wants to hang up a "photograph" of Mira Datar so that she can perform the *loban* ceremony at home. Finally Tajinder will be placed on the large set of scales in the courtyard before the tomb and have herself weighed publicly in foodstuffs, such as grain, flour, sugar, spices or vegetables. Wealthy merchants also place money, silver and gold and a richly embroidered cloth on the grave, which is then handed over to the administrators of the tomb. Tajinder will put on an amulet from the saint for one last time. We wish her well. When we arrive at the tomb the next morning from our hotel in Mehsana they have already left. Their quarters have been rented out to other people.

"Her hair is buried beside the village pond," an old gossip tells us. "Watch out that you don't turn into a *churäl,*" I hiss at her, annoyed that she has divulged the spot, and continue on my way.

A man is circling the dome above the tomb of the paternal grandmother, the Dadima. I have rarely seen a man doing this, and certainly not up here. I wait until he has finished, when he approaches me and says: "I have had my hair cut off. There was *bhut* sitting in it. It is now tightly sealed in a bottle and in the keeping of the *mujawars* down there. It will be buried somewhere or other this evening...," the Muslim, a confectioner, concludes, pointing vaguely into the distance. Tajinder has invented a new custom here, I think to myself.

The Confession

Mira Datar's tomb is a stage, I reflected, and the actors are the spirits which have human beings for their masks.[12] Or are the spirits masks that slip themselves over the people so that they can act? And while I was still pondering over Tajinder, her family and their story, a shrill voice drew me to the women's courtyard and to a new scene.

There a delicately built young girl was resting on her knees and busy screaming out a text, rhythmically and at incredible volume. The voice that was screaming was that of an old woman. It had nothing to do with the petite young girl's body which was writhing there on the stone floor. I was unable to distinguish a single word because I had only just commenced my work here and was not very expert at the various Hindi dialects. If I spoke to somebody it did not mean that I automatically understood their replies. Neither Vikram Nath nor Angana were in eyeshot, so I could not enlist their support. At first I worked only with my old-fashioned Uher Reporter tape recorder, which was a heavy weight to lug around. I still had it over my shoulder because the day had only just begun and I had assumed that there would be a few things worth recording. Yet I was reluctant to switch it on, adjust the microphone and act the part of the well-equipped voyeur in a situation so marked by pain and affliction. But at the same time I urgently required it as a translational aid, as a passing ear, as it were, so I switched it on. Quietly I crouched down close to the girl and set the reels in motion. Her parents, who were sitting beside her, bent over and adjusted her clothing whenever she cast herself to one side and tossed her arms or head or legs into the air. They were the parents of a carefully tended child named Padma who was thirteen years old. They watched over her to ensure that she did not dash her head against the ground or the walls. Every word that Padma screamed seemed to lash her parents like a whip and did not appear to be from their world. They struggled to understand her.

Padma must have kept screaming for quite some time. My tape, which was not switched on at the beginning, recorded almost fifty verses of a text that was certainly many times longer. Later, as I played the tape to S.H.Vatsayan, one of India's leading authors and the editor of the daily Hindi newspaper *Nav Bharat Times*, he was so overcome with emotion that he printed it without any further explanation in a Hindi version under the title "Dark Tales of the Uncanny". What Padma screamed was as follows:

1. "O Lord, my Death, my utterly irrevocable Death, O Mira, reach out to me today, O Mira
2. O Lord, my entire life is already annihilated, O Mira, a life of 45 years has been destroyed, O Mira
3. O Mira, I did not give the sinful blood, this sinful blood, O Mira, to anyone to drink, O Mira
4. But today, O Mira, I was given blood, Mira, I was given blood to drink from the crematorium, O Mira
5. O Mira, today I was given the blood of a black dog to drink, O Mira
6. O Mira, all that is left for me today is a pale skull from the crematorium, O Mira
7. O Master and Emperor, I have nourished eighteen people
   O Kings of Kings, the world of six people has been destroyed
8. O Mira, the life of eighteen people has been destroyed
9. O Master, you have made me unworthy of my life
10. The life of your petitioner is lying here before you, destroyed
11. O Lord and Emperor, you have completed your destruction
12. O Lord, the life of a seeker
13. Destroyer of the life of a petitioner, O Mira
14. O Lord, I am destroyed, O Mira
15. O Lord, the whole household, all are destroyed, O Mira

16. O Mira, the girl who brought in thousands of rupees for you each day, O Mira
17. O Mira, today this girl is destroyed
18. O Lord, today everything is destroyed, O Mira (lengthy repetition)
19. O Lord and Emperor, O Mira
20. O Allah of Medina
21. O Mira, if you order me I shall swear by the holy Koran, O Mira
    (lengthy repetition)
22. O Ali, my Lord,
    this is the conspiracy of all conspiracies, O Mira
23. My destroyed life, O Mira
24. I am 35 years old, O Mira
25. My name is Yashwant Dargarkar, O Mira
26. O Ali, Master and Lord,
    the number of my room is three..., O Mira
27. Ulhasnagar is my village, O Mira
28. O Mira, my home is in Goa
29. She, too, must remain with me for 24 hours ..., O Mira
30. It is now 22 years, O Mira
31. That is how long I have worked in prostitution, O Mira
32. Even today every girl can be had, O Mira
33. They are sold for 50,000 rupees, O Mira
    (repetition)
34. O Lord, O Ali,
    I confess I have already worked in prostitution for 22 years ....,
    O Mira
35. O Mira, I cannot stand
    your conspiracy any longer
36. O Master, the son
    of my destruction has caught up with me, O Mira
37. The son of a bitch has captured me, O Mira
38. Now you have recognised the son of the petitioner, O Mira
39. Now you have seen me, O Mira
40. Now you know the extent of my prostitution, O Mira

41. Which has now been going on for 22 years, O Mira
42. My money is deposited in a bank, O Mira
43. Each girl was sold for 50,000 rupees, O Mira
44 And like the girl, the money as well, O Mira
45. My hundreds and thousands of rupees, O Mira, burned in a fire, O Mira
46. You have brought me to my death, my final death, O Mira
47. O Lord and Emperor, today you have brought me to the moment of my fall, O Mira
48. Time and again I had to drink today from your filthy water, O Mira
    (repetition)
49. Today my death will be final, O Mira
50. Today I shall be put to death, O Lord ..."

The tape ended here. While the text of the individual verse was screamed out in a shrill, screeching voice, like a staccato sprechgesang, the "O Mira" that concludes virtually every line came in a soft, almost singing voice. "O Mira" appears to be the refrain and not a term of address. "O Mira" appears to be Padma, her own voice and not that of the old woman. All of those who later heard the tape agreed on that. Even though there is nothing clear-cut about this story. After playing the tape that evening to Vikram Nath and Angara I asked Vikram Nath what it was about.

"What is that for heaven's sake"

"Padma is possessed by a certain Yashwant D...," he answers drily. "He is a pimp," he adds and gives a bloodier grin than usual, for it's betel nut time, "that much is clear."

Vikram Nath tackles the issue from the practical side. Angana's eyes open wide. Her horror is written all over her face. At the end of Padma's scene I was able to show the two of them the whole family: the small, petite girl who is still a child, and her parents. Angana has the child in front of her eyes and can still hear the voice of the pimp who has entered Padma's body as a *bhut* or *balla*. She is appalled.

"She is possessed by a really bad, nasty spirit," she says slowly, and with that she pulls a blanket over her knees. The next day she says: "I'm going to stay in today, we've still got a lot of tapes to transcribe."

Angana is clear in her mind that Padma is possessed by an evil spirit. And she is unable to gain any distance to this incident. While she was still able to play the objective scientist in Tajinder's case, for that appeared to her to be nothing more than a story that a lot of others had to tell, here she was confronted by a reality that neither she, nor indeed any of us, could understand. The day after I listened to Padma while she talked. Her voice was that of a thirteen year-old schoolgirl, quite different to the one we had recorded on tape. Her family comes from Mumbai. They have come here on account of their mother who feels unwell. But since their arrival Padma keeps falling into a trance. Her parents are worried, and after the occurrence yesterday they are completely beside themselves and totally uncertain as to how to deal with what happened. Everyone knows that yesterday Padma had spoken the confession of an old pimp. Her parents are unable to find any link between any possible eventualities in their own life and what they heard. They are simply unable to comprehend, as indeed are we, how their young daughter could say: "And like the girl, the money as well, O Mira" (verse 44), not to mention such hideous things as: "Today I was given the blood of a black dog to drink" (verse 5). Nor can they make head or tail of this screamed admission of failure from some Yaschwant So-and-so or why, given that it exists, this text should come to be shouted out in public by *their daughter* and not by someone from the appropriate milieu.

I wonder whether verse 48, "I had to drink today from your filthy water," does not indicate that Mira Datar is being addressed directly after all. For if we put ourselves for a moment in the position of a *bhut*, it is clear that it must feel it is being persecuted and driven out and virtually annihilated when it is surrounded by all the trappings of the saint (words, incense, water, shrouds, bangles, horses). A spirit that is in the process of being exorcised sees Mira Datar as his personal destroyer whose (holy) water brings about his downfall. And who apart from Mira could the evil spirit be talking to when it speaks from the girl before Mira's tomb? Padma's case teaches us that we must gradually admit that we cannot always understand everything here. I wondered how long it would take before we all believed in *ballas* or were ourselves possessed by one. It was not to be that long.

The Curse, the Spirits and their Magicians

I have not yet managed to detect the trail that leads to the *ballas* of Tajinder, Padma and the fifteen year-old from Rajasthan. All we know is what people say about it. We have learned that the *ballas* can enter a person when they do the wrong thing at the wrong time and place. We have also heard what the *ballas* say when they speak from their victims' bodies. And we have also seen what they want. We have even heard how it feels when the *balla* rises up inside someone and about what subsequently happens to the person's body. But then the tracks get lost.

I met up with the *ballas* two years later when, one cold January morning, I drove from Delhi and stopped in front of the tomb in order to pay Muhammadhusen and Mazar a short visit. I also wanted to hand them a copy of book (Pfleiderer, 1981) containing an article I had written on the tomb.[13] I was not on my own. I was accompanied by my husband, who had grown curious after hearing about my previous experiences here, as well as by a student from Germany.

Muhammadhusen and Mazar were glad to be honoured by our visit and welcomed us as usual into their office, where they and a number of other *mujawars* were bent over their address lists, writing to clients. I also receive a card from them each year, mostly around the time of the *urs*, the saint's birthday, containing a lengthy prayer and confirmation that they had also prayed for me that year, and telling me that a small donation would help the worship of the saint to be continued in a befitting manner.

Their joy was especially great as they realised that one of the European men "spoke Urdu really beautifully and without any mistakes". They were so delighted that they bent over backwards to tell us the latest news and describe the miracles that the saint had performed in the most appalling cases of deep-rooted possession. "Oh," Muhammadhusen exclaimed, "you must meet the DeSilva family, they've been coming here for years now. They're Anglo-Indians, the husband is a doctor. Come, I'll take you to meet them," he said, and with that he led us out of his office and over to the DeSilvas' quarters.

Mrs DeSilva, a woman who was perhaps in her late forties, received us with a look of expectation in her eye. She was wearing a long, brightly coloured housecoat and was in the process of doing the tidying-up. The family lived like all of the pilgrims in one of the quarters that have been built around the tomb. Not far away their two children were sitting on the ground of the courtyard; both were in their mid-twenties and mentally retarded, as could be seen at a glance. After a while the father, a small, rather unassuming man, came and joined us. He introduced himself and told us that he was a doctor and had practised both allopathy and homoeopathy in Mumbai, but that he was now staying here on account of his family. We asked them whether they would tell us their story and they replied that they were willing to do so. We went and sat in Muhammadhusen's office: the two parents, the three of us and Muhammadhusen. I placed the tape recorder between us and switched it on.

Mrs DeSilva turned to us and began the conversation in English.

"I am certain that you are surprised that we are staying here," she began.

We answered that we were not actually surprised because here a lot of people appeared to be cured of their afflictions.

"Yes, but you must understand that one doesn't generally meet people like us here."

We agreed with them and said that they must have their reasons for being here.

"Oh God," said the woman, "we certainly do, God only knows. I shall tell you about it all."

What followed was an indictment and a self-portrayal that was to last several hours.

"It all began when our neighbour gave our son a piece of

chocolate when he was seven months old," said the father. The child's development took a peculiar turn from then on, he continued, so peculiar that he was forced to believe that his son had a bad character. "He threw things about, acted wildly and would lash out at everything in all directions. But despite this," the father said with a sigh, "I sent him to school, where everything went fine for a while." But then things grew worse than ever. "At about the age of fourteen our son's state was so unbearable that I tried everything, simply everything there was. But nothing helped, regardless of what I tried. It simply got worse and worse. I began to grow indifferent to it all. You see, I'm a Catholic and a doctor, but suddenly I was faced with things that did not fit into my world. On one occasion I went with my boy to a nearby temple, but he got so violent that it took five people to bring him under control. Nevertheless, I tried again at a place of pilgrimage near to us and left him there for one day. When I returned to fetch him he told me that he would come again, see to our needs and then go forever.

He said this and then fell silent for a period of several months. "He lost his tongue," the father said. And once again the father, who was after all a doctor, went from healer to healer and from colleague to colleague. He continued doing so until his wife had a dream:

"Leave your house this evening," she was ordered in her dream, "and go to a great place of pilgrimage, to the tomb of Sayed Ali, and your son will be healed there within three days."

This dream, along with other signs which they listened to, was encouraging them to go to this place here. The dream also made it quite clear though that they should not go to just any temple or tomb, but solely to the main tomb of the Mira Datar cult. The mother was to remain with her son and look after him there. The couple told us that they had now spent almost eight years at Mira Datar's tomb, apart from a few brief interruptions, but their son's health had not improved. On the contrary, it had deteriorated, so that he could now no longer walk upright, look after himself, move about by himself or feed himself. At the same time, when they first arrived here, the father had an attack of paralysis that lasted for six months. Once again the father spoke: "I did my best when my son grew ill. I went to the best doctors in Mumbai. We tried every possible form of treatment."

Up to this point the father and mother had been telling us the story of a sick body. It is the sort of story one would expect from the mouth of a doctor and his Catholic wife. The body was the focus of interest because it was nearing its end, and the main issue was to save it. So one goes from doctor to doctor until one gains a ray of hope. But at this point the story related by the DeSilvas took a surprising turn. Something unexpected occurred.

Let us start again from the beginning. One day the father was sitting with his son in the waiting room of one of the many doctors when another person who was waiting there said: "Doctor, your son won't survive like this." Dr. DeSilva explained this sentence to us, saying: "What the person waiting there with us was actually saying was a pointer to something else." The doctor fell silent for a while, then he looked up at us and said: "That was an indication of something which we call magic, yes, I remembered then," he continued quietly, "that my son had received a piece of chocolate from our neighbour when he was six or seven months old..."

We know this story.

In that moment the doctor must have realised that this new insight was going to lead him to a new reality and to a new way of seeing. The reasons, or the background to his son's declining health were not to be found in the physical realms. The doctor's theories about bodies had become invalid for him. They no longer meant anything to him because the explanations they offered had led to strategies that had become meaningless. He had to turn his back on his medical theories and all of his medicinal categories.

I asked: "What happened to your children?"

At this juncture the mother spoke up and introduced us to the other way in which the matter should be seen: "It got worse and worse, day by day. Our son was chained up here at the tomb and was often locked away because he was so violent. Nothing improved. Because, you see," at which point her voice dropped and she gave us a stealthy look, "it's because they're still doing it. They've even done it to me and made me quite beside myself with rage."

She replied to our questioning looks by saying: "They put a spell, a curse on me. They have put a spell on me with a scorpion," she said, almost whispering. With this she was preparing us for the fact that she, too, had been in trance.

"Who are *they*? I asked her. "One has enemies and they make a contract," Mrs DeSilva replied, "a contract to cast a spell." This statement made the sequence of the events, as seen by the couple, comprehensible to us: the neighbours give the child chocolate, the child's development is abnormal, the father is paralysed for a while, the mother falls into trance.

All that is missing is the information about who made the contract the mother spoke of. I tried a question in order to grope gently after an answer: "Doctor, can you tell me what it means when someone here goes into a trance?" And the father answered: "For me going into trance, or *hajri*, means that one has a personal enemy. That can be recognised by the bewitchment contract that someone makes." At this point his wife interrupted him: "He is only our enemy because we would not let him use our toilet." "Yes," Mr DeSilva confirmed, "the sole reason for all of this is that we would not let him use our toilet." "The toilet in our flat," his wife added by way of explanation.

"You live in a flat?" we asked. And the woman answered: "Yes, we live in a flat in Mumbai. And these people, they live just in a room, and three of them kept using our toilet, and one day we refused to let them. After all, it was our toilet... and we told them they could go and use the public toilet... but we never imagined that they would do something like that to us. I only discovered through my trance," she hesitated, "that they have bewitched me with an African spirit."[14]

"What was that you said?" I asked. And her husband confirmed what his wife had just said: "Yes, a spell from Africa... which she will remain under for the rest of her life."

"Yes," she added, "under a spell for the rest of my life. First me, then our son. From morning till night they invoke an African spell against me."

And the doctor tries to explain to us how it works: "You know, one makes a contract with the spirits that one summons..."

And we, still somewhat astonished by all the turns this story was taking, asked: "And these enemies, do they live in the same building as you?" "Yes," said the woman, "they are our next door neighbours." "And all that," I ask, "just because they weren't allowed to use your toilet?" "Yes," the woman replied.

That was what we needed to be know in order to understand the couple's explanation.[15] The refusal to let the neighbours use the toilet must, as we recall, have come before the chocolate. That is the sequence of events that preceded the calamity that initially came from outside, but now comes from inside.

"They descend on you in such a way," Mrs DeSilva explained, "that you suddenly feel something entering you, yes, something actually enters you. You can feel it. It enters your body and you know where it comes from, you suddenly know who it has come from and then... and it simply brings you hardship and despair."

"What is 'it'?" I interrupted her, to which she replied: "'It' is the evil magic in your body, and everything that was caused by the contract."

And the father: "It enters your body and gives..."

Once again she interrupted him: "Yes, I feel the trance, I feel *them* in the trance."

"And how do *you* feel, what is the experience like?" I inquired.

"I am *outside* of myself."

"And what can you recall, afterwards, I mean?"

"They are inside me and tell me... no, I don't know."

"Does it hurt?"

"You know, your body is overheated..."[16]

Mrs DeSilva no longer feels at home in her body. It is no

longer at her beck and call. She says herself that she is outside of herself, which may be taken quite literally here. She is outside of herself because "they", the evil spirits, *are in her*. They defile her body with their destructive activities. Consequently she no longer trusts her body, it is no longer her own, it has become alien to her: it poses a threat. So she must distance herself from it because it is governed by unknown, alien powers. She now has to watch out for dangers that come from inside of her. The bodies of the mother, the son and also the daughter have been marked, have become victims. More than that, it is the bodies of the people concerned, and just their bodies, that bear the mark of this curse.

It is thus a sensible habit to read from a person's body during the procedures at the tomb just how they and their *balla* are doing. What happens to them occurs likewise in the "countenance of also the body", to use Paul Klee's words.[17] The body is the text of the occurrence. And it can be read to gain directions for further courses of action.

The scorpion magic that assailed Mrs DeSilva made her "forget how to sing and sew", "and even to "overlook the cleaning work". It plunged her into a trance and made her "hair stand on end". She knows that in trance she is turned into a body for those inside her. That is why she loathes trance. Yet she needs it. And the result is the state of helplessness in which she finds herself. During trance texts get spoken that provide the victim with information. They are informed about the *balla's* identity. And simultaneously they learn something about the nature of the contract. Getting to know these texts is the prerequisite for overcoming possession. By using it one gains a vehicle for release.

The father now repeated the technical details of hiring spirits to us in a comprehensible manner. He said, "People who want to contract a spell go to a magician." He is called a *jadugar* or magic-maker in Hindi. At this point the father, who until now had spoken English with us, suddenly switched to Hindi, his native tongue: "The two of them go the cemetery together. And they both have to be naked.[18] Then they summon one of the spirits (he says *bhut*)."

"Do you mean spirits that live in the cemetery and come out of the graves?" I asked.

"Yes, and this spirit is then sent with its instructions... to its victim..." he concluded.

The mother explained the matter further. She said: "You see, it is actually the duty of these *ballas* to punish us. They lash out at my son, on and on until he is completely naked, yes, they tear the clothes from his body! They say as much during the trance: 'We have been sent to do this to you.' And do you know, they keep on playing with the intimate parts of your body. It's embarrassing for me to have to tell all this to you."

Because as we know, only people like sorcerers are naked. Their son has got mixed up in dubious company.

"You can see for yourselves what we have to go through. It's ghastly. We are under a curse. We have gone through the worst experiences you could imagine. Life has become meaningless. It is senseless to do anything else."

The attempt alone to discover the name of the evil-doers had kept them alive. But now they have succeeded in that. At an early point in time they sent their son to the tomb with a nurse, they told us. When they arrived somewhat later they were received by the *mujawar* who had assumed the case, and who told them: "I have important information for you." And after saying that he began reading out a list of names.

"They were the names of our neighbours. We were so utterly appalled at this revelation that we fell into a period of despair," the couple said.

"How did you come by these names? we asked them.

"Their son spoke them while he was in trance," the *mujawar* answered for them.

"Our son was a tiny child when the story began, so how could he have known the names?" Mrs DeSilva asked the *mujawar*.

"It's his *bhut* that speaks when he is in trance," the *mujawar* reminded her.

Two things astonish us here: it is the women who enter a speaking trance at the tomb. The men practise the silent counterpart, *ghum hajri*, the silent trance. We have also seen this at other shrines and I have reported on it in the previous chapter. The fact that the son had spoken in trance not only amazed us at first, but also his parents, because it had not been mentioned until then. And — I would risk saying this evaluatively — no one would have expected as much after seeing him sitting in the courtyard, staring into thin air.

But in this section I am simply reporting what was captured by my tape recorder, and that was what Mr and Mrs DeSilva told us.

"Your son said all that in trance," I asked in astonishment, "although he does not even know your enemies, your neighbours?"

"Yes, he gave all of their names, as well as the motives that led them to perform this deed. And the *mujawar* wrote it all down in his notebook."

At the end of the conversation the parents withdraw to their original world. The father: "The worst illness in the world is the one that is brought about by magic. All that remains is to go to mass and pray with a rosary."

And the mother: "Even during the long years while my son was ill, I never forgot to go back to Mumbai for the major festivals and to decorate the altar at our church. That was what our congregation wished."

But she also had decorating plans for this shrine: "Once my family is well again I shall sew a shroud. It will be red and green because those are the colours they like here." And she would also pay an annual visit, regardless of whether that was the right or the wrong thing to do.

The world into which this married couple withdraws, their world, covered over the abyss which they were just this moment sharing with us. The wife who enjoys singing and sewing is asked by the congregation of her church to decorate the highest of the high, the epitome of purity, the altar. Certain holy days in the church community belong just to her. Her husband, the confidant of numerous patients, enjoys a certain prestige as a result of his work as a doctor. But the children's devilish illness, which is probably constitutional brain damage, and the way they deal with it, shakes the social position they have attained. Consequently their first reaction is to go from "one doctor to the next". But gradually, as the children's fate becomes increasingly clear, long suppressed anxieties work their way up from the (abyssal) depths to the surface: worries about where they belong to, their identity. The guilt and the sequence of events comes to be located in the irrational. The reasons for the occurrences are not perceived by the mind, but by the body. And everything that happens comes from below: the spirits come from the grave and enter the body through the lower orifices — just as a scorpion stings from below and behind.

The story related by the DeSilva family shows me the trail that leads to the *ballas*, to the *bhuts*. None of the foreigners' questions had been left unanswered. We drove on, the atmosphere in the car was quiet and pensive. Our thoughts attempted to exorcise what she termed a curse. I am reminded once again of what Mazar once told me: "The spirits can be recognised by the fact that their footprints are deceptive, for they point in the reverse direction."

Was I on the right track? Our own experiences with the *ballas* were yet to come. Let us return to the story in which we were to get entangled with them through our field work at the tomb.

The Female Anthropologist's Dream

There was a restless feel to the morning. As we will remember, Angana had remained at home in order to transcribe some tapes. She did not want to approach bodies possessed by spirits that day. We went without her to the bus stop where we caught our bus to the tomb. I was feeling uneasy because a dream had alerted me to an inner sense of insecurity. The Indian Government requires that foreign researchers acquire a research permit; a tourist visa expires after only a few months. The research permit I had been given only allowed me to collect data for my project on the Indian film. Obviously our work here at the tomb, which I was doing "on the side" had precious little to do with that. The spirits that appeared to me during my dream told me this in no uncertain terms:

"You're a permit dodger," they accuse me.

"That must be something like a fare dodger," I think in my dreams.

"We're not joking," they reply.

I adopt a respectful attitude towards them. There are three of them. They have forced their way into my hotel room and are standing in the doorway. I am lying in bed and feel that I am at their mercy...

"What did they look like then? Who were they?" the others asked me in the bus as I began to tell them about it all. I started to laugh for I saw that spirits were no less clever than dreams of this kind often are: "They were perfectly disguised. They were wearing trenchcoats and checked scarfs, and each of them was holding a black hat in his hand." They had manifested in such a way that I would take them seriously, and it worked. They said: "If you ask just one more question at the tomb we shall expel you from the country. One more question and that's that!" they said before slamming the door.

I woke with the impression that the door was shut. Only once, when I was drinking a cup of Nescafé at Sardarji's did I feel the urge to think about work again and carry on. Vikram Nath grinned and remarked dryly: "Your spirits!! Nice to make their acquaintance." And Hans, who had trained as a psychotherapist, said in his profound German way: "Oh yes, interesting, very interesting, we shall interpret it this evening."

Unfortunately, we never got that far. It all got lost in something that required far more urgent interpretation. My dream was merely the announcement of greater upsets.

A Drama: Concerning Bees, Ethnographers and their Spirits

On reaching the courtyard of the tomb we sensed a restlessness that struck us as new. The courtyard was like a beehive in which the slightly raised pitch of the buzzing is trying to warn the intruding bee-keeper that the bees are ready for the attack. During the previous days we had conducted a large number of interviews, sometimes each on his or her own, and sometimes together.

Above all Hans had conducted, with Vikram Nath as interpreter, a large number of interviews with the women who fall into trance, as well as with their husbands or families when they were there. These were akin to psychoanalytical interviews, and not always totally in accordance with the indigenous notions about relationships between men and women. Evidently Hans and Vikram Nath had asked married couples about their relationships with one another and then investigated how this related to the problems that had brought them here. For people with a middle-class German background, the idea of linking the quality of a relationship with an illness or disorder has become a normal, everyday thing. Therapists may even dissolve marriages, for in the West the individual has precedence. The relationship comes second.

"If you don't terminate this relationship," as a therapist in Europe may say to a client with impunity, "you will get ill. Only a person who is clinging to a neurosis will stick to an unhealthy relationship," is yet another of the hundred commandments of couple therapy.

Clearly Hans had not managed to make the jump to India, the leap into a society which attaches greater value to the maintenance of social relations than to the preservation of the individual. For Indians in arranged marriages, the notion of separating themselves from their spouse is as out of the question as the idea is to us of divorcing ourselves from our children when they create problems. We do not choose our children, yet we love them "despite everything" while they grow up in our midst. In addition to not choosing their children, the Indians do not choose their spouses, and hold them perhaps "despite everything" in regard. The relationship between marital partners often remains a purely objective one, which tends to have a stabilising effect. Hans, as we were about to find out, had asked too many questions about marital issues. With that he had brought to consciousness things that otherwise remain perfectly suppressed and thus do not cause any disruptions. His questions had led to a great feeling of uneasiness. While Irmtraud, the psychiatrist, often helped me in my explanations with her discreet yet careful observations and what were, as she herself said, often guesses at diagnoses, such as "the young boy there seems to be suffering from hebephrenia" or "the woman there is a borderline case", and all without upsetting the dynamics of the forecourt, Hans had let loose a dynamic process that none of his respondents could cope with. This dynamism now turned against us.[19]

We went and sat down with Shamimbai, who was staying at the tomb because of her daughter Subeida. We had all listened to her on a number of occasions and assumed—quite wrongly, as was shortly to become obvious — that she shared her sorrows with us. Just the day before, Subeida had got involved in a situation that Shamimbai felt was very degrading and unsettling. People had made started making fun of her daughter while she was in trance, and both the mother and the daughter had felt very hurt. She felt robbed of that special space which is essential for the process that the sufferers have to go through here. And she also felt unsure of herself.

"Because," she said, "it is bad for my daughter when people feel entertained at her expense when she is in trance, and not least it shows a complete lack of respect for the two of us. Just look how clean I am here amidst all this filth. All the things one had to take upon oneself," she railed, "but this is the last thing I'll try in the hope of curing my daughter."

We had sat down with her because we already knew her slightly better than the rest and because we felt at ease with her. The day before she had told us that her daughter and her daughter's husband had eaten from a bewitched pan, and now she said that this morning Subeida had vomited one of the pan's nails.

"You won't understand that because you are unable to do so," she said, finishing abruptly.

The three of us sat there in front of her, looking at her, the tape recorder and a camera at our side.

"Not even scientists can get to grips with that," she tried to say in a normal voice, but then something happened to her. Her eyes gazed upwards, no, they rolled upwards so that the whites could be seen. And suddenly she threw herself forward, sending her white *dupatta* flying in the same direction, and her body began to quake. She hurled herself rhythmically against the stone ground of the courtyard and uttered in a hoarse but loud voice — in a holy rage I would say, now that I understand the content — the following curse in the form of a poem, which took up fifteen minutes of tape:

"Not even the scientists win, here we are all slaves to the Lord,
Lord, do not detain me any longer, Emperor and Lord,
They come here and demand miracles, Lord,
And are insatiable, their thirst, Lord,
Is insatiable. Their thirst produces new craving,
Lord, give me the power and the strength that I need, O Lord,
to put them in their place with my word,
O Lord, Sayed Ali, Lord and Protector over this court and this place,
The feeble-minded blatherers,
Who are standing around in front of me,
These doctors of science who have come
To cast doubt on Allah's wisdom, to look behind His order,
O, Allah, their minds are full of science,
Even though no one, O Lord, can attain your miraculous power,
O wonderful Lord, O worker of miracles, drive them away
From my door, these crazed dogs
Who do not understand your power,
O Datar, time and time again you send these devils here to me,
Whom I shall not grant another thing, not another conversation and not even another word.
They throw light on us and research and question us, grill us the whole day long,
And think in the end that all of us here have gas in our heads!
But I say to you, Lord, their heads are full of gas, blood and heat!
Truly they believe just one thing: the problems stem from marriage,

Lie in the marriages of these people here. This makes them suffer and turns them mad, that is what these scientists here think of me.

If you, O Lord, do not keep these roaming spirits in check, then the world is in a sorry state.

Give me, O Lord, the command for me to speak to these shameless people,

These doctors of science who for four days keep coming and standing in front of my door.

They will experience a miracle from me, I shall open

The door of your miracles to them, O Lord, before which the rich bow low,

Before whom Kings place their crowns, before you, O Lord,

None can withstand you, O Lord of Miracles, Saviour of Gujarat,

Show these mad dogs their place, teach them to honour you

And, O Lord, see that they depart.

It remains for you to give the command, O Lord, I have no instructions from you to reprimand them, O Lord,

How did we come to deserve this? I, a mother,

Have scarcely enough time left to worry about my innocent daughter,

She is waiting before your door, even all the *jinnat* respect those who do good,

Not even rogues may be killed without your command,

Our hands would burn if we rose against you, most wondrous one,

They have come to usurp your power of one hundred and twenty-five years standing,[20]

Drive these bloodhounds of science away, Lord,

I am boiling, Lord, I am boiling with rage, no one will be able to calm me any more today

Destroy their brains, Lord,

Their presence here is intolerable."

While Shamimbai was screaming this out, more and more

people came and gathered around us. The men smirked, the women grinned.

"What did she say?" I asked Vikram Nath.

"Well, she didn't exactly given us a warm welcome," he replied, and when I asked him whether she had really called us bloodhounds, he merely said:

"And more. Wait until this evening and we can translate the tape together."

The crowd afforded us protection, separated us from the insulted woman's wrath. We retired. While we were making our way to our rooms Mazar appeared at our side.

"I don't know what's up today, it doesn't seem to be a good day today," he said to us as we left the courtyard in a somewhat despondent mood.

"You can't do any more interviews today," he said, "the atmosphere is too charged. Why don't we take a look at the other buildings at the tomb? You haven't seen anything like all of them," he suggested, and sent for one of his numerous nephews who would act as our guide.

"You could visit the tower, for instance, from there you can view the whole complex. And," he added with a slight grin, "you know the story."

He narrated it to us because Hans and Wanda had not heard it before. I recalled my notes from my last visit here. The story has two parts.

First of all there is the history of the buildings.[21] The ruler Khanderao Gaekwar of Baroda felt that the tomb of the saint, Mira Datar, should be honoured. The rather inconspicuous mausoleum, which up until that time at the middle of the last century had simply been surrounded by a small number of graves and a cemetery, was fitted out more magnificently by the ruler. Around the tomb itself he erected silver railings mounted on silver posts. It is to these silver posts that the red threads are knotted that "tie" the fates of the clients to the saint over the duration in which they "bind" their cure with the tomb. Gaekwar also donated the water tank which nowadays plays the same part in the healing process as the gully that previously occupied the same place in the grounds.

In addition, the outside walls of the entire complex were strengthened and reinforced. This is where the pilgrim's quarters are now located. And the tower also replaced a predecessor on the same site: a post. The post and the gully had a specific function in the ritual process.

While exorcising the evil spirits, the person in question had to undergo certain "punishments" during trance before the demon would leave them.

"And what were the punishments like?" one of us asked.

"You see them being carried out here every day of the week," Mazar replied.

The punishments have not changed, just the buildings. The first punishment which is most frequently "prescribed" is circling the dome of the Dadima, the saint's maternal grandmother.

Probably the second most common punishment is lying down in the sewage water.

"Yes," Wanda said, "I saw that being done here in front of the gate! A woman was lying face-down in the outlet from the toilet. She lay there and the people told me that she had to do this for many hours as a form of punishment, until her *balla* departed from her. I had hoped I had misunderstood what I heard," she added.

I could also recall having seen the same picture on a number of occasions. And I had also hoped I could "overlook" it, take it for a bizarre exception.

"Yes," said Mazar, "those are the people whose *balla* is so impure that the only possibility for them is to pay like with like. But normally the punishment of "lying in water" can be carried out in the tank.

The third punishment consisted of circling round the post, which Khanderav replaced with the large tower.

That brings us to the second part of the story, which in some ways is connected with our presence at the tomb. The post was called *sulli*, a word that is also used for gallows and the act of hanging someone. The punishment that was "prescribed" by the *balla* was likewise termed *sulli*. The victim underwent his punishment within this semantic field revolving around capital punishment. The erection of the tower has changed nothing of this, neither the punishment nor the name. The tower is referred to even now as *sulli*. Nowadays, the pilgrims say they chase the exorcised spirits back to the cemetery, bury them, or send them up to the *sulli*. They repeat this like a refrain.

I was plagued by moments of doubt. Should we climb up the *sulli*, on that of all days? Wasn't that what Shamimbai wanted: "Remove the scientist dogs from my door"? Why had Mazar suggested this to us on that day, when he knew what the atmosphere was like? Why had he grinned when he suggested this to us? And while I was still pondering the matter, Ahmad, his nephew, arrived to take us up the tower. We deposited our equipment and baggage in our room, locked it up and followed him to the tower: Wanda, Hans, Vikram Nath and myself.

The tower is located directly beside the water tank. The door is set in the wall more than a metre above the ground. We climbed up a set of well-worn steps to the door, which Ahmad unlocked for us. It swayed back with a creak, revealing a darkness which we, clambering up behind Ahmad, were reluctant to enter. The air was musty and we could not see a thing. We climbed up several flights of stairs that ran up along the edges of the square building and finally, at the very top, a little light shone in through a skylight. Wanda was climbing behind Ahmad, followed by Hans, then Vikram Nath and myself. Just as I arrived at the skylight and was about to lean out and look at the complex from above, Hans and Wanda came rushing down the flights of stairs, followed by an enormous din from an invisible source.

"Bees," Hans shouted to us, "whatever you do stay where you are," he called as he dashed past us to the exit. Hot on his heels came Wanda, a swarm of bees trailing behind her long, blond, curly wafting hair like a royal entourage. Wanda shouted at the top of her lungs and I thought, My God, us as well, and was about to follow her but she had already vanished. She had leapt from the door one metre above the ground and covered the two metres to the water tank in order to land in the water and escape the bees, which had already taken hold of her hair.

Hans attempted to get rid of his bees under a tap. He was in a bad state. While Wanda succeeded in brushing off her "evil spirits" in the tank — a large number of which were still floating on the surface — Hans had received a large number of stings which had already begun to swell as Vikram Nath and I arrived down below. There was no alternative but to visit a doctor, because stings like these have to be treated with a shot of calcium. We drove off to Mehsana in the car in which we had come, and there took a motor rickshaw to the first dispensary that was open. Hans was administered a calcium injection and sent back to the hotel. I took a rickshaw to Unava in order to spend the evening there. When I got out and approached the gate of the tomb, I found Subeida and her mother Shamimbai sitting on a set of stone steps near the entrance. I looked at them.

"Did the spirits in the *sulli* hit you hard?" Shamimbai asked compassionately. She smiled.

"Hans is in the hotel. The bee stings are really hurting him," I said, returning her smile.

"I would like to listen to your tape," Subeida said to me a few days later, "I don't think that all that my mother said is true."

We listen to the tape that evening. Angana's "Oh God", and Vikram Nath's grins are the first reactions that we receive. Then they translate Shamimbai's words sentence for sentence. We feel intimidated, and a growing sense of shame. The *mujawar's* protection had given us a sense of freedom and led us to feel entitled to conduct interviews with people who had come here because, after all, they felt they were being pursued by an evil party, were possessed by a spirit, or harassed by adverse circumstances. These people were already caught in a hopeless state, which the trance ritual at the tomb was supposed to bring them out of, so our questions had merely exacerbated their distress in a way that no amulet could help. Shamimbai's words had expressed her powerlessness and inability to defend herself in our presence. By saying this in trance she bestowed upon herself the power which she otherwise attributed to the saint. She became his speaker, her curse had ex-cathedra quality. Her sentences became important to us. Whereas our minds are simply "filled" with knowledge, the saint simultaneously "is" and "has" power and knowledge. With her "outbreak" of revulsion at the "bloodhounds" of science who penetrate to the centre of the mind, Shamimbai had spoken a truth which provides an explanation for the cult of possession in its entirety:

She speaks of the threat posed by a different kind of knowledge. She speaks of a knowledge that is alien to her culture but which, as she sees from both herself and from us, leads to a certain kind of power. She realises that it is possible for one form of knowledge to penetrate another and fears that what has been "true" till now will be ousted.

The Enlightenment here in Europe also brought about an "epidemic" of possession cults. These "demonic crises had a double function," writes De Certeau. "On the one hand they showed that the culture had lost its balance, while simultaneously they accelerated the way the culture adapted to the new requirements."[22] (De Certeau, 1980)

Shamimbai's trance was aimed at correcting our behaviour, which was felt to be too importunate. But apart from the embarrassing nature of the accusations, they were also important for the growth of our understanding. It was the only trance text that we acquired that was not connected directly with a healing process that was not spoken under the shadow of an evil spirit. This text said something about the collective anxiety that is felt at a place which is not only a meeting point of the boundaries, but simultaneously a place of retreat. Shamimbai had spoken out and defended herself. She had defended this place as the meeting point of the boundaries and the space it offered.

Later I asked her: "Do you go into trance?" She was sitting before her door and smiling. "Not *napak*, just *pak*," she answered. Not the trance of the demons, but of the saint, she was saying.

Our presence at the tomb had become an imposition. We

had been sent into the *sulli* like the evil spirits the people here try to get rid of. We had lost our sense of balance. One of us had received a swollen body from the bee stings. Another had been seen as she jumped screaming into the water and then boarded a rickshaw dripping wet, her clothes transparent, in order to drive home. We had been marked. As we departed from one another that evening, Vikram Nath said to me, quietly and with a smile:

"Has it occurred to you that we weren't stung by the bees?"

Yet we too had been marked by the *sulli*. When we returned a year later we were greeted by several of the *mujawars* at the bus stop with: "Oh, the people who were stung by the bees have returned!"

The Goddess and the Human Sacrifices

Since none of us wanted or was able to go to the tomb the following morning, Vikram Nath suggested we take the day off. He looked round for a car that would act as a taxi for an excursion.

"We'll drive to the shrine of the goddess Bahuchara," he announced.

"Who is she?" Wanda asked.

"She is sacred to the eunuchs and transvestites who we call *hijra*,"[23] Vikram Nath answered, and he took us to where the hired car was waiting.

After almost an hour we arrive at the goddess's shrine and cross the stone slabs of the large inner court to the temple. Set before the entrance is a small shrine in front of which a large — by Indian standards very large — white cockerel has its place. Although it is neither locked up nor on a chain, it never leaves its pedestal. It is the sacred animal of the goddess, as we are told by the man who looks after it. We can tell from the representations of the goddess that the cockerel is her mount. She looks down from the altar inside her residence, the temple, riding her cockerel with a challenging look. We feel intimidated because she looks down from above. What is challenging her, I wonder, and then leave the temple to walk around the grounds.

"Ha, look, one of us!" a coarse voice cries out.

I look round. Sitting on the shady side of the temple are three women in saris who are pointing their fingers at me. They are shaking with laughter, loud and raucous like crows.

"You're one of us aren't you, show us!" another of them shouts, swaying her hips lewdly. And while she does so two of the women lift their skirts high enough to make the scars they bear from castration clearly visible.

"My God," I mutter, "they're castrated men, *hijras,* who everyone fears but at the same gives money so that they will also bring them luck."

I was about to say: "No, I'm not one of you" when all three called out in unison: "Come on, show us what you are, show us what you've got."

I felt ashamed. This is the worst insult that can be imagined in any culture of the world. I left because the three women, no, men, the three *hijras,* had deeply insulted me: they had exposed their (mutilated) genitals. So even in this inner courtyard I was simply a source of disturbance, someone that people were rude to and called filthy names. I've no luck, I thought.

I had already reached the next shrine, but I could still hear their raucous voices following me: "You're not even like your mother, you slut..."

So this was the sacrifice that the goddess on her cockerel demanded from those who worshipped her. They are shorn of more than their hair and skin. They give her the identity they received when they were created, their identity as men. They offer the goddess their penises and more. It is as if they had given up their minds. And from then on they act out the lives of female bodies that have been mutilated. Some manage the transformation quite successfully. They grow breasts, and if they are emasculated at an early age their faces also remain smooth. But in some cases their bearded faces contrast awkwardly with their enforced femininity. The next shrine tells the legend of this place of pilgrimage in pictures:

Two friends, both kings, swear to unite their children in marriage. But the two only ever sire daughters. Finally the seventh daughter of the one king is declared to be a son on birth and brought up correspondingly. The wedding night reveals though the truth of the matter. Yet the "prince", who is an astute girl, comes up with a ruse in the nick of time. He announces that he will go swimming in public and then present himself to the council. No sooner than he (or she) has said this than he leaps on to his horse and leaves the ramparts, walls and town behind. That evening he arrives with his mare and a bitch that has followed them at a small lake, on the banks of which the goddess Bahuchara is worshipped. The bitch dives into the water and returns to her "master" as a male dog. At once the prince sends the mare into the water as well, and the "test" proves successful. "I shall follow her," "he" thinks to himself and leaps into the water. "He emerged from the water," as the man in the shrine tells us, "in the prime of manhood and returned to the town. The goddess, the ruler over the location where this occurred, merely demanded that he build her a temple and relate the story. We are not told though when she began to demand the reverse from her victims. Like everything that is of duration, this also happened beneath a tree, which is still marvelled at and worshipped in this shrine.

Thus the goddess helped the kings to unite two kingdoms through their children. But for this she required a "miracle" — or victim? — of this kind. And every Hindu man knows what he owes the *hijra* who has no space for himself, neither among the men nor the women, and no function, either as a man or as a woman. He gives the *hijra* alms, a little money in order to keep him at a distance. He pays him off for keeping his distance so that he can maintain his space out there on the boundary. And through their sacrifice the *hijras* are transformed victims, who make up for the aggression and dangerousness of the phallus through their offering to the goddess (Basu, 1993). That is the reason why they merit veneration.

"In point of fact they are in a pretty bad situation, almost like demons," I say to Vikram Nath while we are walking to the exit. "They are people in bodies that are not their own. Or people who no longer have their bodies. They wear their bodies like masks." Masks that give them the possibility of appearing sometimes like men, sometimes like women, and sometimes like spirits.

"And the territory they roam about is constructed exactly the same as their female bodies," he answers. "Their territory is unknown to women, for traditionally women only live "indoors", at home, and only leave home twice: the parental home when they marry and the conjugal home when they die."

"And even death is different for them," says Angana. "They are not allowed to be buried, cremated or laid out for the wild animals or birds the way the Parsis are. And their bodies are only covered in rags when they are brought to the place where the final rites are performed."

Bahuchara is also a place that reveals and celebrates the boundaries, like the tomb.

"A place that teaches you the meaning of fear," says Hans, "and opens up abysses. Abysses of man as a cultural entity and as a cultural animal," he adds, "abysses of the essence and power of culture."

"You can see here the way culture opposes life. I already had enough problems with a God who demands that a father sacrifice his own son, as with Abraham and Isaac, or who allows his own son to be murdered, but here...," Irmtraud says softly, "here people create a goddess for themselves who symbolises and demands reversal, inversion, perversion... and what's more protects it."

"Up till now," says Vikram Nath, "no one has investigated what exactly they do when they sacrifice their manhood. Or where they do it. Perhaps in one of these shrines here."

On the way back home I try to picture to myself the altar on which the victim is placed during the ritual. Does the goddess devour it when she finds pleasure in the sacrifice, does she spit it out when this is not so? We do not want to know or even hear about it.

The Punishments: On the Reversal of Time

After the day we spent visiting the goddess Bahuchara,

we returned to our work at the tomb. We had decided to desist from asking any question whatsoever that might be regarded as impudent and that would simply increase the distress at this place. We wanted to restrict ourselves to having questions asked of us and listening to stories.

Mazar had told us about the punishments to which the pilgrims who have become victims of possession have to submit themselves. All that happens to the pilgrims at the complex is done in accordance with the order of the tomb. More precisely it is a system of ordering time and space. The demons who have entered the victims' bodies have upset the latters' social space and cultural time. The order at the tomb represents the pilgrims' cultural order. The demons that reside in their victims have upset the order of the body. The body no longer houses the person's soul, but rather a demon that destroys order. With that the body loses its balance, becomes over-heated and falls ill.

During the victim's trance the demon, which is holding the body under its control, divulges information on its origins, its identity, its role and its intentions. Consequently the trance is a part of the "cure" at the tomb. Without trance it would be impossible to identify and fight the demon.

The various demons are rated differently.

As we have already heard, the *churäl* is the ghost of a woman who died during pregnancy and, not "knowing" that she is "dead", is unable to find any rest. It is viewed as extremely resistant to exorcism. A woman said to me: "My *churäl* asked me to forgive it during my *hajri*." To which the *mujawars* said: "She must now perform *chauz*, she must now go into the water tank."

The woman had to lie in the water tank until a snatch of dream text or a snatch of trance text advised her whether or not the *churäl* would soon be willing to leave her body in peace. Other women who circled the dome of the Dadima, the maternal grandmother, told me they had to do this as part of the exorcism, which is to say as an action against their churäl.

The people at the tomb also have a clear picture of the

"technical" origins of the demons. We were told that the *farishta*, the angel of goodness, sits inside a person's right shoulder. This part of the person dies after their physical death upon the dissolution of the body through burial or cremation. However, a person's soul or *atma* outlives their death and departs from the individual's body and identity. Consequently this "eternal" dimension of human existence does not get entangled in the demons' affairs. Seated inside a person's left shoulder is evil, the *shaitan* or Satan. After sudden death following an accident, epidemic, suicide, murder, birth or child-bearing, this aspect of the person remains caught up in the individual's everyday life. It is unable to detach itself from the world and from the departed's social surroundings. The result is a ghost which roams about and attempts to enter the body of a close relative. The people at the tomb term it a *balla*. We have come across such a ghost in Tajinder's case. And Mrs DeSilva had explained to us how this *balla* — which she called *jadu* — then enters the person who is designated as its victim in the bewitchment contract.

Another category of demons, named *palit*, also consists of ghosts. They receive particularly harsh treatment at the tomb. They are exorcised by sitting, among other things, in the sewage from the latrines, or by drinking filthy water. As we remember in Padma's trance text, her *balla* complained that it was forced here to drink filthy water. This punishment is called *mori*. Subeida told us that one of her *ballas* came from a very low caste, so the *mujawars* had recommended this punishment in order to drive out the spirit.

"Luckily not the really severe form," she said, "where you have to lie with your face down."

It is said at the tomb though that the hardest punishment is *sulli*, circling the tower, which is recommended in the most stubborn cases of possession. And *sulli*, as we have already noted, is also the word which the judge pronounces when sentencing someone to death by hanging. The victims circle the tower and dome of Dadima when they perform *sulli*. They walk both clockwise and anti-clockwise. All of the punishments inscribe a new pattern in the body: a distance from one's own self. It is as if the victim of possession wants to divert their attention and forget themselves, and to draw the spirit's attention away from them. Anyone who walks against the hand of the clock, like the women here at the dome of Dadima, who often do so day after day at a fast pace, walks out of themselves, steps out of time.

They step out of themselves spatially, just as they step out themselves physically when they are in *hajri*. They leave themselves when they perform their punishments. A woman who is lying head down in the latrine undergoes a hard struggle with herself. She will marshal the totality of cultural and physical force against herself in order to separate herself from what she calls a *churäl, palit, balla*, etc. By means of these practices she will also separate a part of herself which she also terms *randi*, meaning old, depraved whore. This is also one of the categories of demons. A woman who has allowed a space inside her body in which a being of this category could make its home becomes alienated from the time in which she lives. She is no longer "here and now" but in a different time, the time of the demons and she-demons. This now determines her orientation and direction. And we recall what Mazar, the *mujawar*, said: the demons leave footsteps that point in the opposite direction. They reverse both time and order (Kapferer, 1983).[24]

The reversal of the relationships is dramatised on the physical level by vomiting objects that had played a part in the bewitchment contract. The Hindi word for vomiting makes this reversal particularly clear, for it simply means "turning inside out". The body is trying to undo matters when it vomits up the evidence for the contract. The ritual is aimed at undoing matters when it confronts the demon with its demonic reversal. When the victim walks against the direction of time it deprives the demon of its possibility of remaining in cultural or human time. When the victim walks in the direction of time — for hours on end in the burning midday heat — it is trying to brand the cultural time into its body, for it wants to win back this time in order once again to be able to acquire a space within the nexus of cultural, meaningful action. In addition to the punishments comes the trance.

"The end of *loban* ceremony heralds the time when Mira Datar's punishments begin," the *mujawars* say. "The incense drives out the evil spirits, but in some cases it whips up the people and they enter into *hajri* or *ghum hajri*."

When a possessed woman enters into trance her breathing "runs off" with her. It gets faster and faster, until she hyperventilates. Her consciousness leaves the stage of everyday life and she only takes in the actors of her world on the periphery, on the horizon. Her body registers the transition from everyday life to a consciousness of "being-out-there", for it feels a pressure or cold shiver all over its skin. Her body is in pain, torments her; the women often whimper when they "cross over". They only start to emit loud screams once their everyday consciousness has been shed, once they are "outside." And then in trance she can cast off this thing that has got hold of her like the devil: as Padma did with her curse, and Shamimbai with her denunciations, or Subeida did with one *balla* after another. The demons or spirits rise up inside them during trance: they reveal themselves, are *hajri* or "present". As a result of the change in their breathing, their normal, everyday consciousness has been diminished, has disappeared or been almost forgotten. It is not present, and if it is then merely on the fringe, as an objective faculty of memory. What is present is that which has come from outside. But here at the tomb this never results in a journey into a different state of consciousness or into the depths of existence or the infinity of the universe, for it is always the evil, the root of the troubles that appears: sometimes as an image, sometimes as text. And trance also acts to reverse the circumstances.

"I see long-haired black men when I am in *hajri*," Subeida tells us. "They have teeth like vampires."

The demon appears as a mask for the person involved and speaks through her. It is not she herself who speaks. In trance she is not "all there", is literally not herself. She dramatises the Other, the demon who torments her. And through this dramatisation of the demonic she makes the demon present — yet also powerless, because now it must submit to her terms which, as the demon "knows", will end up with it being exorcised from her body. The women say that their body feels heavy and pulls them down to the ground when they sense the trance coming. But once they have gone through the episode their bodies may feel very light, and they walk away with greater ease, almost as if floating. They have "lightened" themselves of the drudgery that subjugates them when they are in its clutches.

The Contest of the Demons

A woman is circling round the tomb. Asma, whom we call the Princess. She rushes along the outside walls getting faster and faster, singing: "Oh Datar, oh Datar." And while her voice is singing, shrill noises emerge from inside her. But now she sees us and slows down. Once her trance has "cooled down" she comes over to us and takes a place at the edge of the group. Kamla, whom we call the Black Widow, gets up as soon as she spots Asma. And Asma says to Kamla, while looking at her through her white veil: "Come on, go into *hajri* Kamla, let's set our *ballas* at one another!"

Kamla likes to provoke people and stir things up. Her eyes are always directed at others, her gaze never without some intent. She's more than willing to set her demon at Asma, I think, and stage a cock fight between the demons...

Asma, who always remains rather reserved, is possessed by the spirit of a maternal aunt who had once fallen into a well. Asma's mother had taken the small girl along with her to watch the corpse being removed. Asma had never been able to forget the sight of the dead body. Shortly after, she grew ill and was never really restored to health. After being married to a butcher by her parents, she came to the tomb in order to ask for good health, because she had already been in *hajri* at other places. In addition she wanted to pray here for a son.

Scarcely have the two young women gone to the courtyard than their voices grow very loud as they "let their *ballas* speak". A large crowd gathers, and Kamla, who is both physically and verbally aggressive, shouts: "I am a *Rajput*!"[25] To which Asma shouts: "You're lying, you're just a ghost from the cemetery, from a grave, you must be a Muslim! And look how weak you're getting, look at the way you're lying on the ground, because my spirit is a strong one which makes people ill and destroys them!"

Then Kamla does something unexpected: she retires to the door of the tomb and explains: "My spirit is simply calm, not weak, and comes to me in *ghum hajri*.[26] He's not going to fight with you."

At that another woman shouts: "What's up with you, you normally spend all your time in trance and raging storming about, and now all of a sudden you're quiet? How can you of all people say that you are in *ghum hajri*?" she says, getting more and more worked up.

But Kamla or her supposed "Rajput" spirit remains unmoved. She simply keeps on singing: "I've got *ghum hajri* and my *balla* is not weak." With that Asma grows proud and "wins" because "her" *balla* is the "stronger" of the two.

This shows once again, if in a different way to the cases we have seen before, how these girls or young women play with "their *ballas*" in order to draw other peoples' attention to them and manipulate their environment. It reminded us, the observers, of what goes on between the clients of certain therapists when they adopt the latters' vocabulary as a weapon in their own confrontations.

Only rarely did we witness such battles, perhaps on just one or two other occasions. Nor are they reported as such from other centres of this kind.[27] On a subsequent visit Vikram Nath and I did however witness a similar drama. In point of fact we came across it more by chance and never got to know the two protagonists. While the scene that I have just described was more like a game between the two women who were undergoing the cure, in the second case we chanced upon a battle between two families. It occurred after the *loban* ceremony, which in any case is a severe test of the cure pilgrims' composure: in the end, one assumes that one is "inhabited by a *balla*" who feels that its right to exist is being threatened by the incense and the presence of the saint, Mira Datar, that this represents. It revolts, as everyone who is possessed by a *balla* knows. Thus for instance while in *hajri* at the loban ceremony, Shamimbai's daughter Subeida asked Mira Datar to be liberated from her *jadu* (demon). The *jadu* replied to Mira Datar by saying: "You're spitting at me (with incense), so I'll spit back, I won't budge an inch from the spot!"

The battle between the women began one Friday after the *loban* ceremony. The one woman, who was wearing a red sari, had entered the customary form of trance here. Her head was lolling between her shoulders, and she was supporting herself with her hands on the ground. Then all at once she cast herself backwards and rolled across the courtyard. All the while her family remained sitting by the entrance to the tomb. Other women were also in trance and were tossing their bodies up and down so that their hair and clothes flew through the air. This is the normal practice at this time of day, nothing more and nothing less. But then the activities in the courtyard changed. A struggle developed when a woman from a different family group, wearing a yellow sari, started to rage in trance directly beside the woman in red. The latter, still completely in trance, stood up and suddenly lashed out at the other, who was moving in her direction. She lashed out at her encroacher, cursed her, screamed and finally leapt at her. The woman in yellow shouted back, took cover for a moment, and then leapt at her opponent in counter-attack. A person beside me remarked: "The *balla* in the first woman is getting into a real rage now, just look at that...!" It struck me that the spectator was trying to egg them on to fight further.

But then the husband of the woman in red came up to her, seized her and hit her. He separated her from the woman in yellow who, lying on the floor, scolded the other: "She can have them all if she likes, *jinnat*[28] and whatever else they're all called. But I won't stand for it if she comes and starts hitting me! In that case anyone could come up to me and..." she shouted. And someone next to us said:

"They often sit together in the evening during the *loban* ceremony and over there at the Mamusahib, the tomb of the uncle. So why this row?" The spectator continued in his astonishment, as the husband of the first woman challenged the family of the second woman and almost turned violent himself when someone interrupted because his wife — the woman in red, who was still in trance — was regaling the courtyard with words like: "I am a good, holy spirit from Pakistan, I am a Sayed, I'm not going to step aside for this *randi*! She's a slut, I'll make sure that she becomes a *randi*, she'll become a whore! I shall go on a blood feud and bring her and her people to their ruin. Yes, I shall visit them this very night..." she kept shouting as her husband came and rained blows on her.

At that point a number of others intervened, and even several *mujawars* tried to help settle matters. But the protagonists had formed such a tangle of arms and legs and heads and words and shouts that it was some time before the people who were trying to intervene and separate them could reach the heart of the group.

"That's not trance, they're not in *hajri*," said a *mujawar*, at first incensed and then astonished that things had got that far.

"They're putting on a show, that's all they're doing. For as long as I can remember people have been in *hajri* here, but nothing like this has ever happened in the courtyard before, not in all my years!"

It is that time of evening, *loban* time, in which everything submerges under the incense, and which unites everyone with the saint. The time in which he punishes and pits his power against the *ballas* and all the other evil spirits. The time for battle.

The Battle: the Saint and the Demons

The first time I saw Subeida was shortly before the *loban* ceremony. She was standing on top of the dome of the Dadima tomb, the highest point of the entire Mira Datar complex, circling the peak of the dome in an anti-clockwise direction. Her hair was undone, and she walked with a slight stoop so that she could touch the dome beneath for safety. I took a picture of her when I arrived up there and saw her walking in trance in a circle before the evening sky. Then I lost sight of her in the crush of the *loban* ceremony. The next day she suddenly stood in front of me, neatly dressed and combed and with a chain around her neck and another around her wrist, both fitted with small padlocks.

"You took a picture of me yesterday, didn't you?"

"Where?" I asked, because I did not recognise her.

"Up on top of the dome of Dadima," she explained.

"That was you?" I asked in astonishment because I did not have the impression that she had been aware of anything up there except herself and her *hajri*.

"Of course it was me who was in *hajri*. I saw you take the photo."

"I thought you were in *hajri*, so how could you have seen me?" I asked distrustfully.

I was often to encounter this same distrust. Later, whenever I gave talks on this tomb to all manner of different groups — doctors, healers, anthropologists or others who were interested — the members of audience would always ask:

"How can you tell if it's trance? Could this woman really have been in trance if she could see you? What do these people take in while they are in trance?" Every time I gave a talk on the subject I would be barraged by this or similar questions from the auditorium. And my answers remained incomplete, for they were those of a person who had never experienced it, someone who had observed but never participated.

Emic and etic[29] as we say in anthropology: a person who dives into the topic and researches from "inside" does so emically. A person who counts, evaluates and analyses — who remains "outside" but renders what they are reporting on comprehensible — performs "etic" research. Although I wanted to be able to say that I was performing emic research during this project, at the same time I did not wish to get personally involved in the fundamental experiences of the women and experience altered states in trance. And this is also what I would choose now, must choose in fact, so as not to forfeit the protective status of the observer.

Only later did the issue start to assume personal relevance for me. The telling moment came during a talk I was invited to give on trance and cures in India at a meeting held by a group of therapists for people interested in transpersonal psychology; someone asked me whether I, too, had gone into trance during my stay at the tomb, and I replied with: "Me? No! Not there!"

That was what did it.

And it would not let go of me any more. A workshop led by Stanislav Grof, which was similar to the one mentioned at the beginning of this book, gave me the long-desired opportunity to have similar experiences to those of the women at the tomb. This was done without taking any substances, but it did involve music, so the "conditions" were not completely identical to those at the Mira Datar Dargah.[30] After this experience, I had no problem in answering the question that I and others had posed: "Are the women who undergo the cure and go into *hajri* before the saint really in trance?" Or is this simply a show, as the indignant *mujawar* said after the "battle of the demons"?

It is not a show. And yet it *can* be one. It is the perception of the inner space and external spaces, as Grof has described so vividly in his numerous books. While in trance a person, who is "out there", also perceives the present, the "here and now": as a basic coordinate, as it were, yet often at great distance.

The second question that was often raised when I gave lectures to audiences who had close connections with psychiatry, was: "Aren't we dealing here with hysteria, as in Freud's and Charcot's days?" This question would take us too far at the moment, but it will be dealt with in Chapter VII.

Subeida may — in both senses of the word — have perceived me and my camera as I photographed her. Subeida is one of the young women who have a lot to deal with at the tomb. She does not just have one demon that "rides" her, but many, and most of them are evil.[31]

I wait up above on the dome of the Dadima for her. Two

farmers from Rajasthan wearing *dhotis*, shirts and white turbans are walking round in a circle. They are pulling along a very, very thin girl with a shaven head. They are walking anti-clockwise round the dome under the scorching midday sun. Dauntlessly. The girl, who is perhaps twelve, thirteen or fourteen and suffering from severe brain damage, shows no will of her own and is scarcely able to walk; she permits herself to be pulled round the dome, gawkily. A person is standing beside me, gaping.

"She is very sick," I say.

"The Devil's inside her," she rasps back, "but," she continues, "*baba* will get him, he'll draw him out of her he will," and she accompanies the words she spits out with the gesture of hurling something with her hand.[32]

All the while the farmers carrying on untiringly. They believe in *baba*. They believe that if they persevere with the punishment of walking anti-clockwise in the blazing heat, the Devil will be hurled out of the girl.

"His powers are infinite," the pilgrims say, "who can doubt it?"

While waiting for Subeida, I remembered the duel between the demons that had taken place between her and a young woman named Razia a few days earlier. That was before her mother, Shamimbai, had tried to send us packing. Subeida's hands were imprisoned in chains, although the padlocks are always unlocked when the women entered into trance. On this day Subeida spent hours in *hajri* and it was not possible to speak with her. And her chains remained padlocked. This hampered her. We did not discover the reason why. Her *jadugar*, her enchanter, was a *bhangi*, an untouchable, she disclosed to us in trance. A person who is possessed by such a one has to perform *mori,* to sit in the latrine. This made her — while he was inside her and spoke through her — untouchable, extremely untouchable, such that she was not allowed even to approach the marble wall of the women's courtyard in front of the tomb. Nobody wants to have a person like that near them when they are attempting, with great toil and effort, to cast out their *balla*. And this likewise hampered her. Thus her *balla* spent the whole morning demonstrating its strength and impressing the others with its threats and poses, which spurred on the women in trance in the courtyard even more.

Razia flew through the gate of the shrine into the street, to the indignation of all who saw. Subeida's *jadugar* screamed out of her and said things about the other ballas that had never been said here before. And in a moment in which she was catapulted even further outside of herself and was completely "beside herself", and in which her hair whisked through the forecourt like a black shadow, the others grabbed hold of her and tugged her, first by her veil, then by her blouse and finally by the hair, across the courtyard. With that she became defenceless, stopped and grew quiet. Shamimbai told this to Angana that evening. She sat before her door and wept, saying that with this she had reached rock bottom.

Later, when Angana spoke to Subeida about this day, she simply waved the matter aside and said: "What do I care? One *balla* attacks another *balla, jadu* fights against *jadu*, what's that to me?"

How removed was she from all this? Her distance seemed suspicious, because things are not all that peaceful among the *ballas, jadus* and *randis* that are inside her and that hurl her body time and again across the courtyard. Even the greatest efforts which the *mujawars* and the saint take to destroy *ballas* are unable to impress the *jadu* inside her. As the incense laid its thick, impenetrable coils around her the spirit spoke out loud and shrill from Subeida's mouth:

"You're spitting at me, so I'll spit back!" And later it added: "And even if you throw me 51 times into your tank, I won't move, I won't budge an inch. Whatever you're planning in order to get me out of here it won't succeed, Mira Datar, because I'll set the whole tank rocking before I take my leave from here..."

Subeida spins in a circle as the *jadu* mockingly delivers a parting shot: "What, you want to hold me under the water. Just try it, for as long as you like, but you won't make me drink a single drop of your water, Mira!"

Nevertheless a number of pilgrims reported that Subeida

had lost one of her *ballas* in the water tank. She had got rid of it by jumping constantly in and out, back and forth, which truly made the whole tank rock to and fro. Perhaps it was the untouchable *jadugar*, because that evening Subeida was seen once again in the women's courtyard close to the tomb. And her mother Shamimbai said that Mira, the Lord, had now called her in after three hours of wildest trance.

Subeida is in *hajri* when she arrives at the platform of the Dadima. On this morning the demoness Aischa is active inside her. She has announced her presence.

"When Aischa is in me," Subeida said later, "all I want to do is roll on the ground and dance."

Aischa has already broken two of the padlocks on her chains.

"She is still uncontrollable," says her mother, and she buys a couple of new ones.

Aischa, the demoness, comes from the potter's caste and lives there where Subeida's parents-in-law reside. She veils her face when she appears in dreams. In trance she says: "I am a living witch, you will utterly destroy me with your incense, you have already captured my 53 assistant spirits, Oh mother, mother, let me live, if I die I shall become a *churäl*, my mother's name is Radhi and comes from Kishangarh, I shall leave you and your parents-in-law, my name is Aischa and I am 45, I shall leave you, Oh mother..."

The rhythm is the same as in Padma's trance. There are also similarities in the text. Is there a pattern here?

Aischa alias Subeida rolls about on the ground by the dome of the Dadima. I am only able to catch snatches of the text which she spits out in her trance. Aischa catapults Subeida's body in time to the words that the latter speaks, onwards down the long, steep steps to the Dadima's tomb. The narrow staircase is filled completely with Subeida's noise and Aischa's raging. And then this screaming, raging figure goes over to the water tank and continues in the water. She only first calms down in the evening after the incense ceremony, when she takes a bath followed by a meal.

The story of Subeida, who has already been mentioned

several times in connection with other women at the shrine, is a typical one. She sits with her mother Shamimbai on the steps of their quarter. The two of them are smiling, and together they narrate the story.

She has already been ill now for five years. It began with sleepless nights, fever, headaches and pains in all of her limbs and her chest, as well as colds. Although she was taken to various doctors, nothing helped. "And how long have you been married?" one of us asks. "Also for five years," says Subeida. "Yes, for five years," her mother confirms, "and she had always been so healthy before she married!" she adds. It all began the first time she went into *hajri* and before that had terrible pains in her chest," she continues. "Afterwards she started to suffer from other problems. As it got worse she left her parents-in-law's home."

She returned to her parents.[33] Then the long search began. She had pains in her chest but in trance she also learned about the magic. And during this period Shamimbai discovered that her daughter's husband had married someone else.

"Her life is ruined," she said to us while speaking about her daughter, "yet we tried everything. But now we have handed over Subeida's welfare to the saint."

"I have pains in my heart," Subeida added, "the *balla* only wants my heart. In fact a *balla* always demands your heart."

The first time Subeida stepped foot in Mira Datar's court or *dargah*, she sat down in front of the marble wall in the women's courtyard with the *mujawar* who received her, and together they recited a simple prayer to the saint: "Whatever might be inside of me, oh Datar *bapu*," she said, "whether *randi, churäl, jadu* or *bhut*, send out your horses, *bapu*,[34] be their match and drive them out, drive them out of me, permit me to leave this court without them all."

The *mujawar* tied a length of red cotton around her wrist in order to empower the formula and to despatch the saint's army of horses. Then he tied a second length of the same thread around one of the silver posts inside the tomb. This is the act of "surrender". The saint now "knows" what is to be done. And the horses must also be given their orders. The *mujawar* reaches into his basket which is full of small, brightly-coloured cloth horses, takes out five of them and swings them 25 times round Subeida's head. That makes a total of 125. Later the *mujawar* tells us: "The army which the saint sends out to dispel Subeida's *bhuts, jadus* and *churäls* is thus made up of 125 horses." In the days that followed, when we talked with Subeida and other women, we kept hearing them say:

"I'm fine, thank you, the saint sent out his horses yesterday."

This stage in the healing process is viewed as the prelude to the battle. After despatching the holy army, Subeida is brushed down with a switch of peacock feathers. With that she is admitted to the cure, the cult and the court. Now when she smells incense she can make the *bhut* in her jump, speak or dance. But when she hits out and kicks others, the padlock she spoke of is fastened to a chain and then hung round her neck. "I have two of them," she says to us, and she shows us the chains hanging from her neck and wrists.

"This is necessitated by the many *bhuts* in her," Shamimbai explains to us. "At first she hit out and raged so furiously that no one felt safe with her."

Fitted out with her padlocks and chains and with a thread about her arm, she is dismissed and sent off to the battle and her cure.

And everyone who goes to be healed at the court "wants" just one thing: that the spirits depart from their bodies, their heads and their lives. And yet: the spirits speak out loud from them, saying that they want to stay, won't budge, will spit back. "And then he gives it to them," said Mr DeSilva while we were sitting in the courtyard watching a man in *hajri*. Opposite the sacred grave is a silver wall that demarcates the men's compound, and before which the head of King Mehendi has been buried. "Which king?" I ask.

A *mujawar* relates the legend. He tells of the sultan in Ahmedabad and of his field marshal. And of the Hindu kings who descended on the sultan's country. The threat became increasingly great, Ahmedabad was in danger, only a miracle could save the situation, the *mujawar* relates. Then the sultan dreamt of a boy who was to be married, but who would first become a miracle-worker. And he was told that this was the field marshal's son, whose name was Mira Sayed Ali Datar. He was just sixteen years old, but that did not deter the sultan. He sent for him. The boy was found in Unava beneath a neem tree, where he was in the process of cleaning his teeth with one of its twigs. The youth was so involved in life that he had become totally engrossed in the preparations his mother was making for his marriage. The sultan's envoy demanded that the boy be handed over. He told his mother: "He is a miracle-worker. A person like him has no part in marriage."

The mother, who later received a largish tomb close to the main one, refused to allow the boy to join the army, so the envoy was forced to return empty-handed. She wanted to make sure he married quickly and, to ensure this, she witheld all of his father's letters which were designed to fire his enthusiasm for this sacred cause. But the sultan persisted in his demands. He sent for him once again, and this time the boy obeyed. He dropped his twig, which later grew into the large tree that now stretches out over his grave, and followed the call of his father, the sultan and the cause of Islam.

With that his story became "men's business" and women had no more place in it. The boy led the army from Ahmedabad to Mandu and won the battle. The hero saw the king in the flesh, and pursued and challenged him. Was he going to surrender to Islam or not, he asked him. As the king demanded back his kingdom the boy attacked him, but the king cut off his head. Mira Datar's body continued to do battle, though, even without its head, until the king was slain. Afterwards he appeared to his father in a dream, in which his body revealed his martyrdom, and requested that he be buried under "his" neem tree. The chiefs of the army and his father obeyed. Furthermore Mira Datar said in the dream that the tree would help everyone who was afflicted with incurable or malevolent illnesses. And finally he requested that the king's head be buried at his feet, so that everyone who came to visit his martyr's grave would stand on it.[35]

And while the *mujawar* narrates the legend — many of

them relate it every day in new versions, sometimes it was only the king's hair that was buried near the saint — a man in *hajri* rushes back and forth between the grave and the king's head with his fist raised, screaming but without articulating any words. The worn-down silver step that leads to this "counter-relic" documents the restless rushing about of generations of men and women possessed by demons.

"Do you see the pleasure he gets from kicking the king's head?" Mrs DeSilva whispered to me while we walked across the inner courtyard. "It does him good, that's why he does it."

And the person walks to and fro, back and forth between the head and the grave, emitting a shrill scream each time he reaches the saint's grave and a muffled roar whenever he steps on the king's head.

"He will keep on screaming like that until he's got rid of his demon," she added.

The transfer which the possessed pilgrims perform at the shrine consists of taking in the holy substance or holy presence in exchange for the demonic presence which we have become acquainted with in the form of *hajri*. Although the demonic presence reveals itself through *hajri*, other forms of this presence can be observed. We can recall in this context Shamimbai's remark that Subeida had vomited a rusty nail from the pan which her *jadugar*, the magic-maker, had used when casting his spell. Time and again when we entered the court in the morning our respondents greeted us with the news that the patients in their families had vomited nails, expectorated stones or found a black worm in their spittle. The victims spit out substances, scream out texts and take in incense, drink holy water and dally by the grave where *karamat*, or the holy power, is at its strongest. The proximity to the grave prompts though the demonic to rise anew:

"If you spit at me I'll spit back," one of Subeida's demons shouted as it was brought close to the holy power. It was unbearable for him. The order of the tomb prescribes punishments as part of the exorcism of the demonic presence: evil is used to drive out evil. The holy presence acts through its inversion: one must first walk through sewage (*mori*), death and time (*sulli*) before one can absorb the saint through incense, presence and text.

This exchange is implemented during the cure. The battle between the demonic and the holy presence takes place in the courtyard. We had just been witnesses to this.

Hajri and the Process of Healing

I wanted to get to know the voices which call themselves *balla* or *bhut* and which speak, sing and shout from the women. I noted that the women's behaviour patterns altered radically when an energy designated as *bhut* spoke from them. In an instant their character, indeed their very being was utterly changed. What were these energies? What effect did these changes have on the women? This question dogged me over the years, but without leading me to any answers.

The question is different when the pious are possessed by a god in a temple. In this case we know the energy that speaks from them, for after all the people have invited it into their bodies. But here in the inner courtyard so many differing energies were speaking from the women that the answer remained a mystery.

Unlike many of my colleagues who have done and still do, I am disinclined to say that the women's possession is attributable to a multiple personality disorder. The psychiatrist who travels to Bali has become a classic case in the medical-anthropological literature. I consider it an act of gross ignorance to lump the spirit possession prevalent among Balinese women healers and their clients into this category. If we study ourselves closely, we can see that all of us have various voices which prompt us, act, break out and on occasion even dominate us. We all keep a number of personalities hidden behind a unifying mask, the persona. Indeed, it may even be a cause of acute embarrassment for one part of a person's personality to learn what another is doing.

This thesis of simultaneously extant mental persons within the one and the same social persona has convincingly been forwarded in the teachings and practice of, among others, the

American research team Stone and Winkelman (1989). From their many years as psychotherapists they have developed a technique of self-discovery which they term "voice dialogue". It is their assumption that we go through life under the protection of a pre-eminent personality component. Those components that help us and enable us to cope with day to day life are the motors, the protectors and the controllers. But at the same time there are also the dancers, the dreamers and the poets, who are often forced to lead a shady existence. These are the gentle as well as the coarse components. Depending on the nature of the primary family situation, suitable personality constellations develop within us to form a social persona. This may get us a long way. But there are sometimes crises in a person's life in which this constellation is no longer suitable, such as the end of a relationship or the regular repetition of problems of a similar cast, or even catastrophes.

Often it is the motors or "pushers", as Stone and Winkelman term them, that propel us into an existential illness during middle age. I have studied Stone and Winkelman's work and watched them in practice. Let us take a brief look at a short excerpt from their work with one of their clients.

In the following we see the story of a client whom we shall call Dr. Miller. He is 45, has three sons and a flourishing medical practice which he runs with his wife. His life is filled out to the very last minute, or rather stuffed full of responsibilities. Everything seems to be in order until one night he is brought into hospital after having a heart attack. We see him here during his convalescence.

The following excerpt is from an interview with the part of him that "pushes" him (and that ultimately made him ill):

Therapist: "I'm curious to get to know you, because you must be the part of Dr. Miller that made him become a successful doctor."

Dr. Miller's pusher: "Of course, without me he would never have got through his studies so smoothly, or the stressful time while he was training to be a specialist. It was I that made sure that Miller earned his money and was a success. I find it hard to watch and see how his illness is making him listen to other voices that are trying to persuade him to lead an easier life."

Therapist: "How long have you been in Miller's life?"

Dr. Miller's pusher: "I appeared when he was at school. I used to help him at sport. I didn't want that he lost or became a loser. That's why I'm worried now when I see how he is looking about in life."

Therapist: "What worries you about that?"

Dr. Miller's pusher: "I'm afraid he'll no longer need me and that he'll lose all the esteem he's got, the success he has and even his job if he doesn't have me to protect him."

Therapist: "I can understand your reservations, and I truly rate all that you have done for Dr. Miller. But his life has undergone a major change through his illness, and it would be good for both you and Dr. Miller if you were to think about you relation with each other."

The therapist then addresses Dr. Miller: "How do you view this force which you owe your pushing energy to?"

Dr.M.: "I recognise it as part of myself, but simply as a part. I could now imagine having this part, this pusher outside now, or just visiting occasionally."

Therapist: "Is there some other part that you're now rediscovering inside yourself, now that you've got so much time?"

D.M.: "Yes, I feel a need, a voice inside me..." His voice grows very quiet and his body appears smaller, more fragile than previously as the pusher has spoken form him, "which I think I know from my childhood and which is asking for more time..."

The therapist focuses on this new energy that has appeared and addresses it: "I'm glad that you're talking with me. Miller hasn't paid you any attention for ages, right? Would you like to tell me something about him?"

The therapist calls this voice Dr. Miller's inner child. It says: "He doesn't allow me anything, not even in the evening when I just want to play with the dog. He keeps on butting in on my time and my desire to do things. Just as soon as I sit with the dog in the yard he has to go and telephone and snatches me out of the silence we have just found for ourselves... But now, now we have time, now life is beautiful..."

Astonished by this sentence, Dr. Miller looks up. He has heard an energy speaking from him which he did not think he knew. In his amazement he says to the therapist: "I've never heard anything like that coming from my mouth before."

"Shall we carry on talking with the small, the fragile part of you?"

"Yes," says Dr. Miller, and he returns to the position in which he had contacted his inner child, "yes, I would like to get to know this voice."

Therapist: "How do you feel?"

Inner child: "I'm glad that I'm allowed to be here." And after a lengthy pause it whispers:

"It's so nice, simply being here and being allowed to have time..."

Therapist: "How old are you?"

Inner child: "I'm small, four perhaps, ... I want to play and let time stand still."

The therapist helps the man during his crisis and illness to find other aspects of his persona that enlarge his existing self-image. He realises that he himself has robbed himself of the time which other aspects of him so urgently require, and that it was the pusher in him that led to his illness, the illness of "racing against time".[36]

The work with these energies, which I have tested on myself and, as a therapist, on many others in line with Stone and Winkelman's teachings, kept making me think back to the courtyard of Mira Datar. For that is what I experienced there.

It is the suppressed demonic, diabolic and other such unholy energies that speak out of the women there, because the women cannot allow them to come to word through their official personae. Let us recall the things that Mazar told me that women should avoid in order to prevent themselves from being attacked by an "evil spirit". They were forbidden to relieve themselves at a crossroads by night, or indeed to walk any distance on their own without company or witnesses. Mazar describes the small, constricted square, the cage in fact which robs the women of their freedom of movement. The persona in Hindu or Muslim cultures represses a lot of the women's voices and energies, which thus have to create other means of obtaining justice.

Here in the court they find their stage.

Let us finally take a look at young Nandabai. She had married ten months before we met her. As the wedding approached she entered, much like Tajinder when she was supposed to marry, a phase of violence and disobedience. She hit her sisters, her brothers, her mother and her father. After the wedding, which included her move to her parents-in-law's house, her body was increasingly beset by pain.

"I don't dare move, it hurts me that much," says Nandabai, "I can't even break bread or hand someone the water," she continues.

Already while at home, but especially since she arrived at the *dargah*, she entered into *hajri*. She rolled, danced, span about the court, turned it into her stage, thrashed about and shouted when anyone dared to restrain her. She created space for herself and maintained her hold over it. And she allowed suppressed energies to speak, as almost all of the women do at the *dargah*. When she was in *hajri* she growled at the others who came too close with a deep, almost gurgling voice. At the *dargah* the chaste, young Hindu woman with her parted hair, her plait and her downcast gaze, turned into a growling beast, a demoness that emitted shrill, fearful cries, into a whore who exhibited her body.

At first Nandabai hit her parents and siblings. Then she was married, which drastically reduced her field of action. She moved into her parents-in-law's home; her body became rigid, it hurt and made her immobile. She slept long hours because the resistance she put up to the circumstances that had been imposed upon her had sorely taxed her. Then she entered into *hajri*. In that state she can pull out all the stops, allow all that had been repressed to speak. Energies that had been denied expression till then were given free rein on this stage:

"My *balla* has long, black hair and a looong, red dress," said Nandabai, drawing out the vowel in long (*lamab* in Hindi) even further... "She says `come with me' and tugs me along, and previously she also appeared to me in a dream, this woman, saying: `Look at me, look at me,' and she forced me to open my eyes. `Come, let's go and play,' she said, and she pulled me over to the door. Then I placed grains of wheat under my bed and she never came again," Nandabai narrated.

But she had not really disappeared, because when Nandabai went back into trance she was there again. Her story was not over. Nandabai will still have to deal with her for quite some time.

In order to protect the women's social personas, these energies are given designations like *bhut*, alias evil spirit, or *bhutani*, their female counterpart, as well as *balla*. Or they are termed she-demons, like the dangerous *churäl*, or the menacing *randi* which instills fear in people with its Kali-like energy. In this way the impermissible no longer has to be suppressed. The reaction to the impositions created by the social role can be spoken out when this is done within the idiom of demonic possession.

In the section entitled "The Pilgrims and the Sick" in Chapter VI, I shall examine the differences that can be observed in the behaviour of the men and women in their courtyards, even though both groups describe themselves initially as "ill" or "possessed". Even the psychotherapists who gave their advice in our study group noticed this difference. Almost all of the sick men who came to the shrine were described as having a "psychosis", whereas no clear-cut category could be found for the women. And how could one!

The women in the *dargah* give rein to suppressed energies. They permit voices to speak which could never come to word in their everyday lives. And they do so in a cunning way. They stage-manage themselves, but they lay aside their everyday mask, their social persona is not to be found on this stage. Here it is the other voices that don the masks, the *bhuts* and *ballas*, and with these masks the women develop their private myths. Each play staged at the *dargah* is part of the history of women in India, but a play that could not be written in the official discourse of Hindu and Muslim India's social code. The history of the whores of Mumbai, Ahmedabad and numerous other cities, as appeared in Padma's representation in the section "The Confession", is one such play. Similarly the play about the forsaken woman who loses her chance of marriage is staged here at the *dargah*, in the present case by Subeida. From Nandabai or even Tajinder we learn the true dimensions of the violation and tragedy that lie behind *shadi*, arranged marriage. Tajinder staged gentle resistance, as I have described in the section "The body, its demon and hair: the *balla*". Nandabai staged a parallel version which involved a greater number of scenes of violence.

While the official culture delineates the space for the women and points out the directions, here at the *dargah* they go in the opposite direction. There are no boundaries at the *dargah*, or not at least those of everyday life. The women do not respect the customary way they are set apart, with two exceptions: they never enter the burial chamber, and a woman has never been seen in the men's compound. But they surmount walls, steps, water tanks, fences and gates when they go into a rage in *hajri*. They lie down in gullies, they are conscious of neither time nor modesty. They encounter the looks they receive from men without lowering their eyes as usual, or without hiding their gaze behind a veil. They abandon themselves to an ecstasy that is normally prohibited to them. They are outside of themselves, while their everyday lives tend to make them die inside. Here in the inner courtyard they live out those parts of themselves that would be unthinkable outside. With this they integrate the latent potential of their personae. They do this through the experiences they have with their own selves, or rather with their own self in all its diversity. Beyond the cultural idiom of possession they know — on a deeper, fundamental level that has remained untouched by anything cultural — that they are more than is to be had from their (narrow) social personae.

This experience of BEING in the demonic, in the infernal, in refusal, in dance and screaming, spitting, cursing, backbiting and laughing — staged through the art and cunning of possession — presents the women with an enlargement of their own persona which can produce enormous changes in their self-perception. A collection of demons constitutes a growth in power. These demons are weapons that can silence even the largest family of in-laws. But one should not overstep the mark. Nandabai answered our question about who does the cooking, now that she can no longer move for pain, by saying: "One day I do the cooking and the next day he does it — otherwise he'd simply hand me my bag and tell me to go, just as he nearly did a couple of days ago when I was in *hajri*. When I came out of it he said `don't do that again my woman'..."

The possessed women at the Mira Datar Dargah are inventive. Their stories are entertaining. The women's courtyard is full of them. It is a real stage which puts on a never-ending stream of new and varied plays each day. That is how inventive the women are. They do not say: "It was always that way", or "That's the way it should be", or "That's the rule here". Their game has no rules, but it is full of life. And with that it is not terrible for them when they unleash such unholy energies. On the contrary, by enacting their plays they are healed of the monotony of the constant "That's the way it should be".

But men also use this stage. They however are bound to the rules, for these are the (male) administrators who attend to official business and recite the accredited version of the Mira Datar myth. They say "It was always that way" and perform the self-same ritual day by day, year after year. I shall show how they do this in the following chapter.

Thus the men who tend to the administration of tomb, and their clients, the possessed women, maintain the cult at the tomb alternatingly at different times and with different intentions. The latter play out their private myths, the former present the official myth. The male clients remain, as I shall show, far removed from the stage. They act out neither the official myth of the administrators nor their own private myths — which they lack — on this stage, as we shall also see in the next chapter.

NOTES

1. *Sardar* means head or chief and is used to address Sikhs. The -ji suffix is a term of respect.
2. *Balla* or *bhut* are the two synonyms used in this institution for an evil spirit. The victims believe that their bodies are inhabited by such a spirit. As such they are involuntary victims. This form of spirit possession is regarded as undesirable. When the victims are in trance the evil spirit comes to the fore; it becomes a person within the person, and has its own identity. Since it is the wish of everyone that it should go, they obey the wishes it expresses, which are the conditions it makes for its disappearance. The Western expert on spirit possession, Erika Bourguignon, writes in her book *Possession*, 1976, that a distinction should be made between possession and possession with trance. The former brings about a visible change in the physical functions, such as in an illness. The latter brings about a change in the person and their consciousness during the trance (Bourguignon, 1976, pp. 3–6). In addition she maintains in her book that possession with trance appears predominantly in farming societies, whilst possession without trance tends to feature among hunting and fishing cultures (ibid, pp. 46–47). The observations made at the Mira Datar cult do not support such a categorisation.
3. Mazar chose the term *jinn* here. This term is understood all over the Muslim world and is thus pan-Muslim, as it were. He probably used it here in order to document his membership to the international Islamic community.
4. It is assumed that prior to the appearance of the Muslims, this region contained places of Hindu and pre-Hindu worship in which the horse played a part. Since rudiments of the horse cult can still be found in the vicinity in tribal and non-tribal cultures, it may be assumed that the horse ritual in the Mira Datar cult has very ancient roots. What can nowadays be seen there are the small cloth horses fashioned out of the *gilaf*, the shroud, which are swung across the pilgrim's head in groups of five a total of twenty-five times —making "125 horses" in all. When the *mujawars* talk of "sending out the horses" they mean that the 125 horses form an army. This army of 125 horses is sent out to catch, fight and destroy or simply drive off the *balla* or *bhut*, and at any rate to render it harmless to the victim. When Mazar speaks in the present

context of "sending out the horses" he means that they have also continued hunting the balla during Tajinder's absence, and are performing as it were an exorcism at a distance.

5. Frank Rollier reports in his study on a Muslim tomb in southern India, Murugmalla, that the pilgrims' hair is often offered there to the deity in thanksgiving. The same is also reported from Hindu temples. (Rollier, 1982. p.13)
6. *Na* means not, *pak* means pure. Women are impure when they have their period and are not allowed to enter any shrine, whether Hindu or Muslim, for the duration. During this time they are particularly susceptible to spirit possession.
7. Besides his proper function as barber, the *nai* has another function in society: he brings the news from one family to the next about the appearance, behaviour and state of the marriageable sons and daughters. He knows all the details and can be trusted, and thus is asked for advice when daughters or sons have reached marrying age in the household.
8. *Bol-na* means to speak in Hindi. *Bai* is a suffix frequently appended to first names and means roughly sister.
9. A *ta'widh* is a medium for transmitting holy power. It is an amulet made of the saint's *gilaf* or shroud. A person who wears it is in contact with the power that is ascribed to the grave. The pilgrims and invalids take the amulets that have been made for them by the *mujawars* back home with them.
10. In Chapter II, I pointed out that, in both the Hindu social theory as well as ayurvedic physiology, women bring their "heat" *(tapas)* under control by means of the designated patriarchal order. Too much heat makes a woman mad, said the healer Shastriji. Too much heat makes them uncontrollable, so the fathers of unmarried daughters think.
11. Pilgrims often take an oil lamp full of sanctified oil as well as a consecrated brick back home with them after they have been cured at Mira Datar's tomb. They then found a new Mira Datar cult in their region. These satellite shrines are termed *chillas* (see note 11).
12. Michel Leiris (1958) writes that the master of possession, the Zar, acts like a mask in a theatre: the person becomes the Zar.
13. In this article the function of the Muslim places of pilgrimage *(dargahs)* are described and their tradition and origins examined. Several aspects are explained once again in the present work in the chapter "The Tomb and its Order".

14. The word used by the married couple was *jadu* or *African jadu*. This means first of all magic, either good or evil, and more specifically African magic. The person who does the magic is the *jadugar* or literally the magic-maker. He is sought out by someone who wishes to take the spirits into custody. We were told this time and again by the pilgrims at the tomb. They said that the adversary or evil-doer had hired a magic-maker who gave contracts to the spirits roaming about the *kabarstan*, the cemetery or cremation grounds, to possess someone and harass them or even ruin their lives. The route into the person is often, indeed almost always via food. This explains what the thirteen year-old Padma said in trance about the blood that "she" had to drink, and likewise the way the DeSilvas fixed their attention on the chocolate that their neighbour had given the children.
15. The couple does not have a readily comprehensible status in Indian society: as Anglo-Indians they belong neither to the Hindu nor the Muslim caste system. Consequently their identity is threatened. In what way are they Indians? This may partly be explained by what the husband said at the beginning of the interview: that he is a Catholic and a doctor. Both act for him as a kind of caste system. Membership to both, the Church and the academic world, is tantamount to caste membership. I would interpret their statement that they were victims of an *African jadu*, an evil magic, as a reflection of their threatened identity. Africa stands for them for low caste, for "savage", far remote from any kind of civilisation and pollutive. And their neighbours had indeed polluted by using their toilet. The vocabulary of purity is easy to deal with in India: one remains inside one's caste and adheres to its taboos on purity. If one meets someone from another caste or culture one must minimise as far as possible all points of contact — both bodily and eye contact. The differences of opinions between the neighbouring parties only became dangerous because they concerned the body and notions of cleanliness. This upset the DeSilvas. When they started to be stand-offish this was prompted by fears of a reaction or quite simply of revenge. The problems within their own family could thus be projected on to this causal chain. The augmented form of the African magic is the scorpion magic, for it is even more "savage" and unpredictable and dangerous. Through these metaphors Mrs DeSilva is expressing her feelings of

helplessness. The savageness that descended upon her becomes manifest when she enters trance, when her son sits on the floor unable to walk and plays with his "unmentionables", as she puts it. She is even able to distance herself from this uncivilised behaviour when she refers to it as African magic.

16. Mrs DeSilva is saying much the same here as Tajinder's mother had done. The notion comes from ayurvedic medicine, which says that the body must not get overheated. An overheated body reveals quite specific symptoms, just as a body that has accumulated too much mucous, bile or wind in its system shows other specific symptoms. The harmony of the body is determined by diet, climate and behaviour: these must be kept in balance. If climate or diet has led to an excessive build-up of mucous or bile in the body, the harmony is disrupted and the body displays symptoms. Thus Tajinder for instance was diagnosed by her mother as being "overheated" when she returned at the onset of her illness from school with a fever, so she was given a cooling drink.
17. The title of this book was originally to be "A Countenance of also the Body" after the title of a painting by Paul Klee. The bodies in trance at the tomb create the story, which they narrate to form a "countenance of also the body". Paul Klee's painting greatly resembles some of the drawings the possessed women drew at our request of their spirits.
18. In India the body is not even exposed within the confines of the family. Nakedness is the exception, and assumes a marginal status: the Jain monks of a particular order go naked, as do sometimes sadhus (holy men). When nudity is mentioned here it is intended to underline the monstrosity of the procedure.
19. In the current psychiatric manuals hebephrenia is described as a form of schizophrenia that manifests itself in the young, mostly for a short period. A borderline case is viewed as a mental state close to schizophrenia. I have avoided using psychiatric termini in this work because they are inadequate for describing the occurrences at the tomb.
20. The number 125 means at the tomb approximately the power of the saint. The *mujawars* say that Mira Datar's army consisted of 125,000 cavalrymen. When a patient arrives they send out Mira Datar's army of 125 horses, where the number 125 stands for both his army and his own personal power (see footnote

4). Likewise Shamimbai is referring to both the size of the army and the power of the saint when she says "of 125 years standing".

21. The groundplan of the tomb has been given at the end of the book in order to make this section clearer.
22. De Certeau, 1980, p.8. And one could also say, that the voices of the possessed people are a metalanguage which accompanies traumatic cultural change.
23. The *hijras* are an (unofficial) institution in Indian society. They sing at weddings and dance for the tourists. It is said that they were born hermaphrodites, but this does not always appear to be the case. There are few studies to my knowledge on this group. One of the best known in the West is Serena Nanda's *Neither Man nor Woman—The Hijras of India*. Many of them were presumably abducted or persuaded to join the cult of Bahuchara. It is said that the temple in Gujarat also serves for the act of castration. *Hijras* wear women's clothes as a matter of principle. In the anthropological literature they are likened to the Berdache of the North American Indians, the Xanith of the Arabs and the Mahus in Polynesia.
24. Bruce Kapferer writes in his exhaustive study on the healing of victims of spirit possession in Sri Lanka, *A Celebration of Demons*, that the exorcists say that the spirits and demons represent the reversal of the world and of the cosmic order of the universe. They destroy the cultural aspect of the persona, the ego. The exorcism annuls this reversal when the demons appear on a proper stage before their victims and subject them to a deep emotional shock. The long ritual process of the *Tovil* rite reassembles the personality when the latter experiences a reversal of the order into which the spirits have precipitated it (Kapferer, 1983, p.111). The ritual process at the tomb delineates a similarly reversed order. The victims are cast out of themselves by the trance, by a physical revulsion that exceeds all bounds, and by the ceaseless, dizzying process of encircling the dome or tower. During this process the possessed women attempt to divorce themselves from the voices of the demons and to re-constitute their persona.
25. *Rajputs* are the landowner caste, the *Kshatriyas*, of the province of Rajasthan. Theirs is a very popular caste that many non-Rajputs try to "join" by altering their names. This is viewed as deceit. This "lordly caste" is made particularly appealing (also to tourists) by its legendary feudal, chivalrous lifestyle.

26. *Ghum hajri* is the silent and distinguished form of trance that is practised by the men and rarely by the women. In the eyes of the observer, though, only the "loud", visible form exists. We only found out about the silent trance during our conversations, and as such it remained simply a phenomenon that people mentioned and talked about when they wish to explain the techniques of the healing process. Entering into trance cannot be dispensed with since it is a part of this process. Thus if one is loathe to be seen screeching and wailing in the tomb's courtyards one "declares" oneself to be a "practitioner of *ghum hajri*".
27. Rollier, who has published highly comparable observations on the Murugmalla tomb, mentions nothing of this kind, even though the formal course of events at the tomb, its order and the notions about the body and the demons are in complete agreement with those at the Mira Datar Dargah.
28. *Jinnat* or *jinn* are the same as *bhut, balla* or *jadu*. The former are used in Urdu, the latter in Hindi. *Jinnat* or *jinn* come from the Arabic and stands for spirits that come from the ground (cf. note 26, chapter 3). Here the woman is protecting herself against the *jinnat* as if from an infection; in much the same the way as one might say: "Keep your flu germs away from me...," she is saying roughly: "Don't infect me with your demon!"
29. *Emic* and *etic* are terms derived from phonemic and phonetic in linguistics. Phonemic is applied when language and its components are understood according to the categories used by the speaker, i.e. from the inner standpoint. Phonetic, on the other hand, is used when language is analysed as it were according to scientific practice, as when a linguist, for instance, tackles language purely descriptively and from the outside. This categorisation of the anthropological methods of observation came into vogue during the 1950s. At this time anthropologists began increasingly to use "participant observation" or "observational participation" in order to gain their material. This means quite simply living with the people on whom one wishes to report. Naturally there are differing shades of this somewhat utilitarian form of living together. When working in an institution in which cures are performed by means of trance, the question will arise as to whether the events that one describes can be judged emically — from within — when one merely "lives together" with the people involved, or whether it is also necessary to experience the healing

process, the dreams and trances if one wishes to be regarded as an "emic" observer.

30. Stanislav Grof is a psychiatrist from Prague. He initially experimented with LSD after it was manufactured synthetically by Albert Hoffmann, and later used it in clinical and psychotherapeutic contexts and founded his own school (Grof, 1988). When work with the substance became no longer possible, he and his wife Christina Grof developed a technique they termed holotropic breathing. This psychotherapeutic technique is based on the same technique that is used for "entering trance" here at the tomb and at other temple centres in India. The practitioner undertakes a period of fast breathing or hyperventilation and maintains this rigorously until he or she reaches an altered state of consciousness. In the therapy developed by the Grofs the client is advised to wear a blindfold in order to block out visual stimuli. It should be mentioned though that the breathing is performed to a specific kind and sequence of music. During this process the frontal brain and thus the memory of everyday events slips into the background and the bodily memory is awakened. With this the practitioner reaches spheres of being which cannot be contacted by means of "normal", "hylotropic" memory. Grof is a leading representative of transpersonal psychology.
31. During another study of possession and trance performed in the Himalayas, I learned from the main protagonists — possession specialists or *shamans* — that they perceive the helping spirit or deity that they sense within them as one who "rides" them (see Pfleiderer, 1983b).
32. Many of the pilgrims and patients refer to the saint as *baba*, which means roughly old father, wise one or trusted one. In addition low-caste servants or children are addressed with baba, showing the feeling of trust involved.
33. When a woman marries she leaves her parental home, termed *ghar*, and goes to the home of her parents-in-law, which is called *sasural*. A woman only returns to her *ghar* when visiting. If however she returns once and for all, a thing that is culturally undesirable and only happens as a result of ill fortune, her parental home is now referred to from this new perspective as *maika*. The case described here concerns a young woman who had fallen ill and was perhaps no longer supported by her in-laws, and had then returned to her parents. Many parents refuse to receive their daughters back, whereupon many of

them live a life of often fatal helplessness. Subeida was fortunate: her mother took her "back" to the *maika* and even accompanied her during her cure. This is more conceivable among Muslims because, unlike Hindus, marriages are often contracted within the family circle. Marriage between parallel cousins is common practice among Muslims, whilst Hindus marry their children within the same caste, but outside of the family circle, such that Hindu women become true "strangers" to their own homes. (See: Michaels, 1986 and Pfleiderer, 1987.)

34. *Bapu* means here roughly Oh Lord, Oh Father. It is used as an alternative to *baba*.
35. Historically speaking the saint can be established as the son of Dosan Miyan who settled in Unava in 1463 and married into the Sham-i-Burhani family. His grandfather was Sayed Ilm-ud-din from Unchh, who was chief commander of the army under Ahmad I (1411–1442), the founder of Ahmedabad (Nawab and Seddon, 1928, p.91). The battle that is related in the legends reputedly cost 19,000 Rajputs their lives during the siege of Mandu by Muzzafar II on February 23, 1518 (see also Pfleiderer, 1981, pp. 195–233).
36. Helman (1987) describes how in our culture alone time is a dead, measurable, lifeless mass that is clapped over the physiological processes of the body. Co-ordinating oneself with time is dangerous when one's appointment calendar is over-full. Helman links heart attacks with man's race against time. He shows that if we leave everything up to the "pushers", which is essentially all that this "Type A Behaviour Pattern" is in the end, and not allow other voices that wish to lure us into timeless moments come to word in our daily rhythm, we are running ourselves to death.

Chapter 6

The Men's Stage

Cult and Cure at the Mira Datar Dargah II

Urs: *The Saint's Day*

In early Autumn, after our return home, I received a copy of a printed letter which Muhammadhusen sends out to all of the *dargah* pilgrims. "May this letter reach you in perfect health and with the grace of the Almighty. May you come closer to your aims and have success," it said. And then came the explanation:

"The *Urs Sharif* of the great saint Mira Sayed Ali Datar will be held this year on the 23rd of November. Please let me know if you wish to participate. We shall arrange everything for you. If you cannot attend because of work commitments then send me a money transfer by post so that we can pray for you, bring rose water to the tomb, and buy flowers and cloth for the shroud."

This request is then repeated directly afterwards: "If you wish to send me money, please send it to the address below and give my greetings to all at your home. Yours, in prayer, Sayed Muhammadhusen Valimiya."

I was unable to travel to India in November and thus fell into the category of those who "have work commitments". So I wrote to Vikram Nath and asked him whether he had time to go to Unava during the *Urs* period. He said he could and travelled there.

Muslims in south Asia call the festivities to celebrate the anniversary of their saint's death *Urs*. The original meaning of the word, which comes from the Arabic, is marriage or wedding. The celebration of the *Urs Sharif* illustrates the union of the saint with the divine. *Sharif* means holy, so the wedding here is of a spiritual nature. The saint's relationship with God is often described in terms of the bride who longs for her beloved (Basu, 1993). The saint's life does not end with his physical death, for death simply means a new state for his holiness. He may now act in the proximity of the divine, and can now distribute infinite *karamat* (happiness and well being).

His anniversary is truly his day. His links throughout India's Muslim community become manifest. Emissaries from other cults and other saints come as guests. They come in order to wish him well. It is his time; it is scarcely imaginable that the women would now spin through the court in trance, as on normal days when the saint "does his duty" for others. No, today even the most crazed women join the solemn procession which is held in his honour. The *Urs* is his day and the magnificent display that is put on is in his honour.

Vikram Nath reported to me on Mira Datar's *Urs*. The following pages are based on what I learned from him.

He arrived at 2:30 p.m. in the warm November sun. It was the 26th of November, or 28 Moharram according to the Muslim calendar. The *Urs* was held later than planned. Wooden stalls had been set up along the streets for the sale of devotional objects, souvenirs and food. The pilgrims were already arriving in streams, but the police were also there in large numbers to ensure law and order. A large number of families had already settled in the roofed-in part of the inner courtyard of the tomb and spread out their belongings. It had become almost impossible to set foot upon the ground. The old dignitaries were nowhere to be seen, just the young *mujawars* busied themselves with their pilgrims, their *sawwalis*.

Coconuts were constantly being offered before the saint's tomb. And incense was being burnt at all four corners of the burial chamber while the Koran was read by the wall that separates the tomb from the men's compound. From time to time the customary rhythmic sound of "high-ee-high" rang through the air from women in trance (*hajri*).

It had just turned half past three when the older *mujawars* crossed the courtyard. They opened their offices and began to deal with the letters from their clients, which had been sent to them from all over the world so that rose water, a shroud and petals would be placed on the grave in their name.

Now various groups of fakirs, who had travelled from all over Gujarat, came and pitched their chandarvas, their baldachin-like tents. The courtyard was filling up.[1]

Then the *medni* procession arrived from Ahmedabad, the capital of Gujarat. This is the procession of the flag-bearers or *nissandars*. They arrived at the village at the stroke of three and reached the entrance to the *dargah* at half past, bearing twelve flags. The flag-bearers were followed by musicians playing drums (*dhol*) and oboes (*shehnai*). One of the people in the procession carried a censer. There were forty of them in all.

As they approached the *dargah* none of the *mujawars*, not even the younger among them, were there to receive them. The spectators were surprised at this, but not for long, for scarcely was the procession level with the main entrance than twenty crazed women forced their way into the rows of the flag-bearers, all the while dancing, singing, turning cart-wheels and generally making a wild confusion of the orderly procession, which continued a further four hundred metres to the *mamu-dargah*. Later, at around four p.m., they returned to the entrance of the main *dargah*. The participants went in by the entrance that connects the courtyard to the street, and once inside they were shown to the three rooms that were to act as their lodgings for the five or six days of the *Urs*.

After the five o'-clock prayer, the *asar ki namaz*, the flag-bearers brought their flags out of their rooms. The musicians began to play their drums and oboes. The pilgrims decorated the flags with garlands and kissed them. There were four large flags and eight small, green ones. The number of the small flags varies, for they are donated by pilgrims when a wish has been granted or a vow been kept. The large flags were brightly coloured; three of them were white and trimmed with red and green silk borders. Attached to their tip was a horse made of cloth. The fourth was brightly printed. Fluttering from the tip were additional pieces of red and green silk, along with embroidered silk saris that were donated fourteen years ago by a woman pilgrim. This pilgrim, a *Lakshmibai* from Nasik, had established her own Mira Datar dargah, a *chilla*,[2] and donated this valuable piece of ornate cloth to mark the occasion.

The most important flag-bearer, the one who heads the procession, is also called the *sandal-mujawar*. He wears a white cloak and a green turban, Vikram Nath continued.

Once again they proceeded out through the entrance and down the street to the tomb of the saint's maternal uncle (*mamu*), the *mamu-dargah*, and then back to the saint's tomb via the main entrance. The flag-bearers then attended the evening loban ceremony in the *mamu-dargah*, and only arrived in the courtyard before the tomb at half past six, when it was already dark. They lowered their flags in front of the entrance, pointing them towards the holy grave. First the small flags, which were then slowly furled and placed on the ground at the tomb's entrance so that they came in contact with the *majjar sharif*, the saint's grave. A number of the *mujawars* appeared in the doorway and tried to grab the cloth horses that were attached to the flags. Afterwards the flags were taken to the mosque in the tomb grounds, where they were received by the *mujawars* and placed for safe-keeping in the nagar-khana, the drum house.

As the sun set the number of pilgrims grew. The courtyards were brightly illuminated; every surface was covered with people. Then it was the turn of the four main flags. It took a while before they were rolled up, for they are large.

The pilgrims had come from all over India: from Bikaner, Bhopal, Nagpur, Surat and Mumbai. Many are from the surrounding area. Some come here each year to celebrate the *Urs*, and keep returning as long as they live. Others have come for the first time.

In the meantime the booths have all been set up, over fifty or sixty of them. There must be hundreds of them. The majority of stalls sell food, others sell clothes, and yet others sell jewelery, toys, amulets and coloured prints. In addition there a couple of rifle ranges. There are even two tents in front of the gate to the tomb that act as cinemas where films can be watched, and likewise a theatre has been erected for the occasion, in which up to sixty pilgrims can watch dance and mime. And towering over the square before the entrance is a big wheel and beside this a couple of carousels.

The pilgrims have pitched their tents along the walls of the tomb, both inside and out, as well as in the courtyards and corridors. Some have even erected a kitchen tent, and yet others have built small huts beside the road.

The activities of the possessed women have slipped into the background. During the days of the *Urs* the saint's power belongs to the *umma,* the congregation of the faithful. It is they who spread the tidings of his sacred power across the land in the form of various manifestations.

As the stream of pilgrims continues to swell the mountain of shoes that have to be attended at the entrance becomes so enormous that the shoe attendant now only looks after the *mujawars'* footwear. The courtyard of the tomb is filled to overflowing, there is no space left for another pilgrim's feet.

The owners of the tea stalls water down their tea by degrees, in order to keep up with the growing demand. The people who rent out rooms manage for their part by increasing their prices from 200 to 300 rupees. This is almost impossibly expensive, it's a fortune, a quarter of a teacher's wages.

The most sacred rituals are conducted during the night before the actual *Urs.* This is the most highly charged moment in the inner courtyard and the high-point of the festival.

Originally the "Sandal Ceremony" had been planned for the 28th of November, but since the moon was not visible the *mujawars* decided to postpone it by 24 hours. The pilgrims have handed the *mujawars* their pieces of sandalwood which are then ground down and made into a paste.

First thing in the morning, at around 3 a.m., the *mujawars* set off to the inner sanctum, the burial chamber. They enter through a door that may not be used by anyone but the *mujawars,* the door on the western side facing Mecca. They close the door behind them and begin their ceremony in the tiny, closed and unventilated room. It is very cramped inside and there is very little light.

During the night the flowers have been removed from the grave. The old shrouds have been folded and placed in a wooden trunk by the north-east door. These will later be used by the *mujawars'* families to make the cloth horses which the *mujawars* use during their prayers with their clients. The grave is now completely uncovered. We should remember here that the *Urs* is the saint's betrothal to the divine. Just as the bride is rubbed down during the night before the wedding with *mehndi,* a cooling dye, the saint's grave is now coated with the cooling sandalwood paste. But before this it is washed down and cleansed with perfumed water in a ritual called ghusl. The water is drawn from the saint's well and mixed with extracts of rose petals. After washing down the sarcophagus the used water is filled into containers and later given to the faithful to drink.

Once the sacred bath has been completed the grave slab is covered with sandalwood paste. Each *mujawar* has brought his own sandalwood mixture. The attendants of the sacred grave bend over the stone slab inside the cramped chamber, move their hands full of sandal paste across the slab and begin to coat the stone. They have to force their hands through the crowded bodies to the slab, for there is scarcely room for all. New hands keep pushing their way through the crush to the slab until the entire surface is covered with hands that move about it with a soft scraping sound. It is as if they wanted to do the saint's corpse a good deed by anointing it with the wonderfully fragrant paste.

There is so little air inside that one of the *mujawars* opens the western door and leaves, spluttering. Others throng after him. Once the entire grave has been coated with paste the *mujawars* drape it with silk shrouds donated by pilgrims. After about two hours the ritual inside the heart of the complex is over. The guardians of the sacred power step outside. They have to battle their way back across the courtyard. They push and shove. The crush of pilgrims who have witnessed the sacred ritual blocks their way so that it is almost impossible for them to move forwards. It is now approaching 5 a.m., writes Vikram Nath.

At other Muslim tombs the cooling sandal paste ceremony is followed by the dance of the fakirs, who enter into "divine possession" before the saint. This is a "warming" possession that is supposed to counter-balance the cool condition of the saint. In analogy to this the bride who is kept "cool" at a wedding is brought together with a matrimonial clown who symbolises the "hot" sexuality by means of lewd movements. According to Basu, the possession of the dancers by the saint during the *Urs* is of especial importance to the *Sidis* of Gujarat, a group of former slaves from Ethiopia. The *Sidis* are also known in Gujarat as a kind of fakir brotherhood who appear publicly as ritual clowns or fools (Basu, 1993). As we shall see, they also have their place in the ritual at this tomb and in its *Urs*.

As morning broke a dense, never-ending stream of pilgrims entered the burial chamber from the courtyard, continues Vikram Nath in his report. The pressure inside from the human bodies grew unbearable. The pilgrims inside the chamber had closed one of the doors while others shouted and hammered at it until it was reopened. The restrained, holy atmosphere that had been so full of reverence and anticipation early that morning had been dispelled to give way to a hectic feeling of panic. Everyone wants to touch the grave right at this instant, now, when it has the greatest degree of *karamat*, has been freshly charged with healing power; the pilgrims want to run their hands over it and come close to this source of well-being now, for this is the most auspicious moment for approaching the divine. And because everyone wanted to do so at the same time, pilgrims were sent flying through all of the doors of the tomb and into the courtyard — hurled into the outside world by the pressure build-up from the human bodies inside the chamber.

At the same time the sons of the local fakir group offered the saint's bath water to the pilgrims to drink. It grew lighter. Many of the pilgrims now asked for a mark to be made on their foreheads in sandalwood paste. Some are successful and leave with the cherished sign.

Once the sun was high enough to reach the inner courtyard the fakir groups began to make their entrances and with that show their reverence to the saint.

The first to appear were the *Shah-Madar* fakirs. They had come the day before to the tomb by foot from the village of Lunava, which is situated in the same district. Their religious leader had died a few months before, so in his place they carried a symbolic coconut decorated with rose petals. They expressed their reverence for the saint by means of a simple dance, which they call *dakhol*, around the tomb.

As it turned nine o'clock the Rifai fakirs entered the courtyard. Their leader or *sadar khalifa* strode before them carrying a dangerously sharp-looking iron spike (*gurz*) which is beautifully decorated and strung with iron chains. Scarcely had they have formed a circle in the inner courtyard than the *sadar khalifa* leapt into their midst and thrust the iron spike into his eye. "A horrific sight," writes Vikram Nath, "you feel you can see his eye trickling down his face. And what is worse the leader dances all the while and remains quite relaxed, as if nothing had happened." The others then followed the leader and formed a circle, flaying their necks, bellies and shoulders with chains. It was painful to watch them.

While the *Rifai* fakirs continued their torture dance in the circle the aforementioned *Sidis* entered the courtyard to pay their respects to the saint. Their Afro-Ethiopian origins are not only recogniseable from their physiques, but also from their music instruments and the rhythms to which their bodies dance. This group did not only consist of men, as is customary. No, here everyone sings and dances, men, women and children. Their saint, Bava Gor, whom they worship at their home close to Bahruch in Gujarat, has a sister, Mai Mishra, whom they also revere. She was represented here by the Sidi women, who carried her with them in symbolic form: a coconut shell wrapped in a silk scarf and filled with pebbles, which is used as a rattle while they sing. They call their dance *dammal*, which comes from the Urdu word *dama* and means approximately breath or intoxication. They also call it *ngoma*, which indicates its African origins (cf. Basu, 1993). While they sang and danced, one of them hopped around in the circle and played the clown by assuming all manner of amusing postures and getting up to other tricks. The spectators tossed two-rupee, sometimes five-rupee notes into the circle, which he picked up with his mouth when he had not already managed to catch them in mid-air. Here they play the part of the "natural clowns" that their African origins have earned them. This has brought them into a "between and betwixt" position in the Indian caste system. This role is the frame for their caste identity.

The *Jallali* fakirs said that they would save their performance for the evening. They are weighed down with iron. In their right hands they carry a fire sign. Their waists are girded with iron chains, their wrists and ankles are decorated with iron bracelets. While paying their respects in the saint's courtyard they danced and beat themselves with their iron chains. "That's nothing," one of them said to Vikram Nath, "in the old days we used to wear twelve iron rings each on every hand and foot, but now it's just two or three." After the Jallali group had finished their dance they walked round collecting alms. They have different names for this right to receive alms: *kisti, kichkod* or *gurupatra*.

All of the fakir groups have the right to receive alms from the street vendors' stalls, and mostly they are given bread and lentils. Some of the groups supplied information on their income from the alms: it was not much more than a thousand rupees for the whole group. The fakir groups depart for home three of four days after the Sandal ceremony, leaving behind them a shroud as an offering. The *mujawars* say a prayer for them in exchange and give them the saint's blessing.

All of the fakir groups have the right to stay at a particular place in the inner courtyard during the *Urs*, one that they return to each year. These places bear the names of their respective fakir groups, such as *Jallali-chauk, Rafai-fakir chauk*, etc. This concludes Vikram Nath's report.

The relationship that the fakir groups have to the saint's grave shows the importance and status of the saint in the ritual world of the north-west Indian Muslims. The saint is covered with shrouds that have been donated by pilgrims who have come greater or lesser distances. He is honoured by means of fragrant sandalwood paste, which likewise comes from a great many different regions and households. He is presented with dances and performances so that his blessings will be carried far and wide. During the festivities for his anniversary the saint is offered dances, music, sandalwood paste, and care and attention. He receives the *karamat*, his power and strength, back from those to whom he normally offers it the whole year long. As a result of their offerings the saint's power is put in the pilgrims own hands, just as the people have their sovereignty on the day and in the minute they vote.

This exchange between the pilgrims and the saint maintains the life at the places of pilgrimage and creates the stage for the possessed women.

The *Mujawars* or the Guardians of the House

When I first began visiting the tomb I asked one of the many young boys who can always be found in the courtyard: "What does *mujawar* mean?"

"It means guide in English," he replied.

"And why guide?" I asked. "A guide to the grave, to the saint, and to his *karamat*," the boy answered patiently.

Like everyone here, he named the saint *Datar Bapu*, an expression which has connotations of intimacy and almost tenderness. Later I heard the same information being given time and time again: guide. On returning home I opened the *Encyclopaedia of Islam* and discovered the following entry: "mudjavir ... the term indicates a person who, for a shorter or longer period of time, settles in a holy place in order to lead a life of asceticism and religious contemplation and to receive the baraka of that place. Such places are the Ka'aba in Mecca, *haram* in Jerusalem and the prophet's tomb in Medina, but also tombs of earlier prophets..." (Ende, 1991)

The *mujawars* at the tomb of Mira Datar are far removed from this description. They are the owners of a sinecure which they have acquired as follows: several hundred years ago the *mujawars'* ancestors, who belong to the *Suhrawardi* caste, settled in the region of Ahmedabad. Mira Datar's father, Sayed Dosan Miyan, was the first of the family to move to Unava. He figures in the legends surrounding the saint as the field marshal under the Sultan of Ahmedabad. Some twenty to twenty-five generations separate him and the present members of the family. The *mujawars* at the tomb live from the fact that they are identified with these origins. It is their capital. The *mujawars* immediately show the inquisitive visitor the ancestral line that transforms each of the living *mujawars* at the tomb into a relative of the saint. The saint's grave is surrounded by the graves of people to whom each member of the family can also establish a connection. Generally it is the saint's brothers or their wives and mothers who are referred to.

Since there are no publications on the tomb apart from my own, I must rely on what I myself have seen and heard. In an earlier work (Pfleiderer, 1981) I gave a detailed description of the history and administrative aspects of the *mujawars*' role. I described how the Muslim community first raised objections to the family's sinecures and made sure that the shrine was declared a *waqf*. This corresponds with our notion of common land. The family went to court and spent decades haggling and trying to regain their private rights. But without success. Eventually even the state, which was still under British rule, felt compelled to intercede. Then in 1949 the *mujawars* were told that their shrine was a public, religious institution for the benefit of the community. The saint's family, however, remained resolute. They went to court again, and this time they managed to have the tomb declared a public trust and to secure the hereditary right to administer it. They had to agree though that two outside members would be elected to the administrative committee. That is the present status quo, much to the annoyance of the *mujawars*, for now the state can say that the toilets were never constructed to cope with the current numbers of pilgrims and have to be renewed. If one asks the *mujawars* how business is doing they will reply: "We have had to build five new toilets, even though we never needed them beforehand."

The most serious intervention was doubtless the stipulation

that a designated group of witnesses has to attend the weekly opening of the collection box (*golakh*). The *mujawars* acquiesced, annoyed, but swiftly found a way around this. But they do not tamper with the administrative ritual and thus acknowledge the status quo after their own fashion.

One way of assuring a regular income is to keep up a lengthy list of clients. The clients are regularly requested to attend the *Urs*, to pray and to make donations, as in the letter at the beginning of this chapter. The *mujawars* say that they write to hundreds, in some cases thousands of clients. A young mujawar named Sayed Latif Miyan said that he had written to some four thousand people and that two thousand five hundred of them had responded with a payment.

Apart from this, the *mujawars* also have to attend to the upkeep of the grave. This is expected by the community and by everyone who feels connected with all that goes on at the tomb. In practical terms this means that they must attend to the daily duties at the tomb. The person on duty goes to the burial chamber at sunrise and removes the petals from the day before. He also removes the soiled shrouds and replaces them with fresh ones which he takes from a box specially for this purpose. The lord must be ready to receive all his visitors, as they put it, the day's pilgrims who will bring fresh petals and ask for his help.

If one asks the *mujawars* about all the activities that can be observed at the tomb, they will tell of miracles that the saint has performed, indeed performs every day "because his miraculous power is glorious, omnipotent and omnipresent", as they say, and they begin to give examples.

"Come," they will say, "and see the miracle that he has performed for the DeSilva family." We recall here the story of the mother and father who visited the tomb on account of their handicapped children. Or, "Quick, a girl has been healed. This girl has finally been cured after years of suffering." We recall here Tajinder's ritually shorn hair and *balla* possession.

If one asks the *mujawars* why one witnesses such dramatic histories of affliction and such dramatic demonstrations of possession in the inner courtyard, they will relate how the evil spirits enter the women.

Mazar, the oldest son of Muhammadhusen, told me how this occurs: "If a woman squats at a crossroads in order to attend to nature's call, and moreover is alone, a *balla* will enter her. If a woman is unclean, which we also call *napak*,[3] but still wishes to go to a holy place, a *balla* will enter her. If a woman enters a mosque and her hair is not properly covered a *balla* will enter her..."

Mazar's list seemed never-ending. I stopped him after five minutes because I did not know what to make of his passion for this subject. My tape recorder documented the whole litany. The regulations that he listed make the room in which women are allowed to move so incredibly small that it made me, a mere listener, feel I was suffocating. And yet I had to admit to myself and to the women who live in such reduced circumstances that they master the ruses of the impotent with perfection. They simply let out and give leave to the demon inside of them, if that is the only way out from the narrow path. Thus they also use the regulations that constrict them in order to act freely: the "codeword" is *hajri*, visible demonic possession. And under this guise they can risk saying a thing or two, as we have already seen.

Sayed Miyan Yusuf Miyan is a master of his art. He reveals to me how he wins over clients: "I ask Datar Bapu for dreams, dreams that he sends to our clients so that their attention will be drawn to the Mira Datar shrine."

In addition he uses his own dreams of the clients with whom he is currently working. I ask him whether he really does have such dreams and he replies: "Yes, of course. Just listen to this story!" And he tells me of a case that he had recently come across at the *dargah*:

"There was a young married couple here. They came after having a dream of Mira Datar. We performed an admission ceremony together in which I had them repeat the prayer to Datar Bapu, and tied a red thread around her wrist and its counterpart round one of the silver pillars of the tomb. We performed this outside because the lady had her period and was *napak* (unclean) and could not enter the inner courtyard.

So then I sent out the horses for her, the saint's horse army. It is up to them to track down the *balla* and drive it out. That's why the women go into trance, into *hajri* as we say here. But this woman did not enter into *hajri*."

"So you wanted to make sure that she went into *hajri*? Why do you even think she is possessed by an evil spirit?" I interrupted him.

"The woman had health problems, apart from which the couple wanted a son and did not have one yet. That's a sure sign of a *balla*," said Latif.

"And you wanted her to enter *hajri* so that you could help her, help her with her problem, which is to say help her to acknowledge her *balla*. Only when she has acknowledged her problem, the *balla*, can you help her to exorcise it. Is that right?" I asked.

"That's right," he replied. "But listen to what happened then. The couple only wanted to stay for one day, but I advised them to lengthen their stay because the woman still hadn't entered *hajri*. They then stayed for three days, and during the last night I dreamt that the woman was in *hajri*!"

The next morning he rushed to get to the *dargah* and find the woman so that he could ask her whether she had experienced *hajri*. But the couple had already set out on the journey home and could not be found. Not even at the railway station at Unjha.

"But," he continued, beaming, "three days later they were back again. They had returned! And do you know why?" he asked in a commanding manner.

"I think I can guess," I replied. "Yes," he said, "they came back because the lady entered *hajri* when she got home!"

"You see," he continued, "that is our task. We have to lead our clients to a place inside themselves that helps them to gain clarity. That is why we call ourselves *mujawars*, guides."

I was impressed by the Latif's conception of himself and his work. After this conversation I viewed the *mujawars* as distinctly more than simply the fortuitous owners of a family sinecure. I had gained a feeling of respect, even though the matter with the bees should have made me realize that the *mujawars* who were dealing with us had also developed a clever theory about us and our own dynamics.

Latif continued his lecture: "You see, when a woman is in *hajri* she says things you would not otherwise find out. She tells us who is responsible for her having a *balla* or *bhut*. If we're lucky she names the *jadugar*, the magician who cast the spell on her. We've had cases where the magic-maker was so clearly described that the victim could return to her village and verify the matter. With that everyone involved was able to get a clear picture of the process that had brought about the calamity."

"Is that the objective of this process of clarification: confronting the magic-makers with the truth and taking them as it were to task?" I asked.

"No, the aim of the process here is to make the victims realise what is happening to them and what has happened. Only then can they escape their wretched state and perhaps avoid getting into a new one," he replied.

"How does *hajri* occur?" I asked. "It is brought about by the saint's miraculous power," he replied briefly.

"Another part of our duties," he continued, "is our work with dreams. The pilgrims come here so that we can interpret their dreams. We have also experienced real miracles in this connection, because we have also been able to discover the reason for the magic from the dreams. We call this magic *jadu*. We listen to the dreams and then give our opinion on them. That's why people come here," he concluded.

Ahmed Ali, the brother of the *Sajjadanashin* Muhammadhusen, also talked about his work with dreams. He told me about a woman who had already spent forty days at the tomb without anything starting to happen. She had originally made the pilgrimage to the saint's tomb on account of persistent stomach complaints. She was hoping for an improvement but nothing occurred — until she had an experience in a dream.

Ahmed Ali said: "In her dream she saw an uncommonly handsome young man wearing a face mask. He told the woman that he would operate on her. He had the same instruments that one sees at a doctor's. He told the woman to remove her clothing from her stomach and she obeyed, and then he operated on her, removed a large, hard substance from her stomach which we call *goth,* and sewed her back up again. When the woman woke up she saw the magical stitches on her stomach, and she was quite astonished at them because there was no one in the vicinity who could have done such a thing to her. That same morning she came to my brother Muhammedhusen and told him her dream. He said to her: `Be grateful, my daughter, Datar Bapu has just given you a great boon. He has taken away your complaint. You may now return to your home.' This woman now has six children, is happy and content, and has remained healthy ever since. She comes to the tomb each year to attest to her devotion," he said in conclusion to his story.

Ahmed Ali explained further: "We can recognise the patient's condition in our dreams. When we dream that the pilgrim is sitting in a train we know that they are about to be healed. When we dream that someone enters or leaves the tomb or is travelling through the countryside we know that he or she will soon be restored to health. A transition of this kind indicates that they are about to return home."

Another *mujawar*, Sayed Umsali, explained to me how he combines the mailing business with his dream work. He said that he receives some seven hundred letters before the *Urs*. The majority of them contain money and the request for a prayer. He said that when the instructions are not sufficiently specific he prays at the tomb for the client ten to fifteen times, just as his colleagues do. "Give the pilgrim who cannot come in person a *bascharat*, a dream that will help them to reach the right decisions," he prays. Umsali emphasizes that this prayer is answered in "75%" of all cases.

"And what rules do you use to interpret your clients' dreams as well as your own?" I asked.

"In a bad dream you see the snake," he replied, "in a good one you see green plants. The dreams are like films. Even if you can't understand the words you know what is up with the patient and understand their problems."

What the *mujawars* convey to me here about their conception of themselves reminds me of a term we use in medical anthropology: therapy management group.[4] And indeed, the *mujawars* give constant advice to their clients during their stay at the shrine and thus have a fundamental effect on what occurs in the courtyard.

This realisation prompted me to take another look at the *Encyclopaedia of Islam*, and there at the end of the entry on "mudjavir" I discovered the following sentence: "In more recent times the term *mudjavir* has gradually become used to indicate permanently-appointed personnel of places of pilgrimage (guards, cleaners, guides ...) who in general belong to the local population." (Ende, 1991)

The part played by the *mujawars* at the Mira Datar Dargah fits this final entry in the encyclopedia. They come from a local group which legitimates itself by means of kinship to the saint of the tomb. They maintain the place of pilgrimage and are at the same time the clients' guides during their un-holy episodes.

The *Sajjadanashin*

"He who sits on the prayer mat in worship" is the literal translation of this title. Sayed Muhammedhusen Valimiya held this title at the time I conducted my interviews at the *dargah*. According to the official genealogy he belongs to the twenty-sixth generation that is descended from the saint's brother. The forty to sixty *mujawars* who attend to the clients at the tomb acknowledge him as the ritual and administrative chief of the institution. All of the *mujawars* have the same background regarding descent, so evidently there must be other prerequisites for gaining the office of *Sajjadanashin*. Piety or money? I suspect both in his case. The majority of the inhabitable buildings in the vicinity of the tomb belonged to him; his biography reveals that he was present at the *dargah* at an early age.

I was told by a woman colleague that the struggles at other various *dargahs* over this office look much the same as those in any political contest: intrigues, lies, defamations

(Jeffery, 1981). Muhammedhusen, who died not long ago at the age of seventy, never spoke to us about his office and power. Perhaps that was the best stratagem. Instead we simply heard him talk about what openly occurred at the *dargah*: the miracles, the cures, the stories.

Naturally he was also one of the few remaining witnesses to the institution's history. Already in 1940, when he was just 21, the elders of the shrine used him to win one of the court cases against state intervention.

The ethnic and social make-up of the pilgrims was completely different at that time than it is now. Nowadays anyone will come who can afford the bus or train fare, which means that the tomb is also visited by thousands of people from the lowest and poorest castes. This was not possible in the past. The pilgrims were, as he told us, mainly from the middle classes and the upper strata of society. Everyone had of course to make their own sleeping arrangements, because the pilgrims' quarters did not exist then: the courtyards were full of ox-carts, horses and camels. He also told us of his work with the clients, how he interpreted dreams and recited prayers. "If a dream is full of foreboding for the patient we will only tell them if it will help the cure," he said.

"How does one become a *mujawar*?" I asked. "Oh, everybody in our family can become one." He himself had tied a length of the *chilla* round his wrist and the remainder round one of the pillars of the tomb at the age of nineteen. With that he documented to himself, his family and the community that he wished to work as a *mujawar*. He worked his whole life long in the *dargah*.

All of the *mujawars* with whom I spoke told me that they had learned to interpret dreams, attend to their clients and administer their address lists by observing the older *mujawars*. One simply has to be there all the time and one learns how to do the work, as the majority of the people I asked told me.

"What does a *mujawar* do when he himself receives a hard knock?" I asked Muhammadhusen. He fell silent and studied the floor.

"Once, many years ago, I was at my wit's end," he replied

after a brief pause, "Mazar was dying. We first fetched four doctors from Unjha, and then another from Palanpur. Mazar's stomach was enormously distended, his intestines were about to burst, and he had fallen unconscious. We had spent an enormous amount of money and now the doctor told us: `Your son will be dead within six hours.' I kept watch the whole night long. At three a.m. I recited a prayer from the Koran one hundred and twenty-five times. I must have fallen asleep afterwards because then a dream came to me.

"I dreamed..." he broke off here and began to weep softly, "that Mira Datar came to me mounted on a horse and said: 'Have you completely forgotten me during all of this?'" The *Sajjadanashin* now began to weep bitterly, but he continued his story:

"Datar, my Lord, said to me: `Bring your son to me, dip the four corners of the shroud in water, wring them out and give the water to your son to drink, and then take him back home.'

"I did as I was told. I took my son to the courtyard at the break of day, asked someone to open up the burial chamber, dipped the shroud in water, gave this to Mazar to drink and took him back home. I cried the whole time. Once we were back home my son at once fell into a deep sleep. After a whole week of nursing him we also fell asleep, exhausted, and only woke up again at 8 a.m. The boy was still asleep, but the wind in his stomach had diminished and his pulse had returned to normal. I called a government doctor and told him to distribute all his expensive medicine among the poor; he told me that my boy was healthy. The next night Mira Datar appeared to me in another dream: he moved his hands over Mazar's stomach and said: `Put your mind at rest and give him *gilaf* water, the water from the shroud, twice a day.' Which I did. After two weeks my boy was strong and healthy. After six months we had him married."

He smiled, and even now one could still see his relief.

"What did Mira Datar look like in the dream?" I asked.

"I did not see his face because he radiated so much light it hurt my eyes. So all I caught sight of were his feet. His feet were of such untold beauty that I could scarcely remove my gaze from them."

After Muhammedhusen had finished his story we remained for a long while sitting in silence. It was evident that he needed to free himself once again of the emotional shock he had undergone back then.

"What was it like with the possessed women in those days?" I asked after a while. "These stories of bewitchment are new, or at least to this extent," he answered. I picture to myself a courtyard in which camels and horses were housed, and which was none too suited to what we could observe during our talk, and think: "In that case the possessed women of Mira Datar are something new, something that is happening now and that does not have a history."

In the villages from which the possessed women come one can find *bhopas*, possession specialists who beat the woman with chains until the *bhut*, the evil spirit, leaves. Or they suck it out of the sick person's stomach or scratch their clients' skin with a knife in order to prompt the spirit to flee. On one occasion I spent an entire week sitting next to a *bhopa* and watched him at work.

"No, there have always been possessed women, or for a long time at least," I replied to the *Sajjadanashin*, "but the stage that they have created for themselves here is new, as is the play that they have developed here in your courtyard."

"Yes, that's right," he said, adding with a grin: "we have become a kind of `mass medium' for possession here."

The Pilgrims and the Sick

Of the pilgrims and the sick who come to the tomb, it is only the women and not the men who transform the inner courtyard into their stage. One has to look around the courtyard for some time before one finds the men. Although the courtyard is full of *mujawars* and their relatives, as well as all the many small boys who have nothing to do at home and amuse themselves by watching the continually unrolling performance here — one does not see any male pilgrims or patients at first. One only discovers the male inhabitants behind the *mujawars'* office block after taking a walk round the complex. They live in a small courtyard and the majority of them are chained up, because their stories are quite different to the women's and tend to express themselves in violence. There is no movement in this courtyard, a rigidity prevails. They stand along the wall with their chains around their wrists or ankles. The majority remain silent.

A small boy aged about fourteen greets us with a raised hand. "I am a policeman," he calls to the visitors and gives us a salute. Our psychiatrist has examined him. "A case of hebephrenia," she tells us after she has studied him and his history. She explains that this is a form of schizophrenia that is encountered among adolescents. His story was as follows: one day he refused to take part in anything at school. He was taken home where he began to beat his sister. When he started to reach for pieces of furniture in order to hit his parents, they were forced to tie him up. For a while the parents kept the boy at home with the family, but then they had to take him to a doctor because he threatened to run wild. The doctor explained enough about the psychiatric nature of the illness for them to understand why he required in-patient treatment. The parents were afraid of this, though, because it would damage the other children's chances of marriage, so they looked for another possibility. With that the boy arrived at the Mira Datar Dargah.

The men stay in the western section facing Mecca, which is obviously the better part of the tomb if they want to be close to the saint. One of them found satisfaction in walking back and forth for hours each day between Mira Datar's grave and the wall of the tomb, which contains the Hindu king slain by the saint: he walked forwards to the grave and backwards to the King's head, which he stamped on each time he reached it.

"It really does him good," Mrs DeSilva said to us when we first arrived at the tomb. "It really does him good to stamp on the king's head."

Another of the inhabitants was something of an exception among the men. He said that he had an evil spirit inside him who had been a sword-dancer. As for himself, he was simply a taxi driver from Madras, but the spirit was a Rajput or landowner from Rajasthan. A sword-dancer, as he also called him, who had built thousands, or more precisely 23,000 locks inside his joints, for which reason he had to dance all day, sometimes on his feet, sometimes on his head. We were sitting in the men's courtyard by the tomb as he told us this. He had already been dancing as we arrived that morning, and he was still dancing as we left in the evening. One could almost believe that one could hear the locks rattling in his joints.

Sitting on the steps before the tomb was a young man. He was almost thirty years old, a Muslim, and we tried to ask him which region he came from. His wrists were bound with black chains and his gaze was generally directed upwards at an angle, as if following an invisible trail in the air. We sat down beside him and talked with him.

"Where do you come from... from which town?" one of us began, and with that he unleashed a torrent of words which we thought would never end. The following is taken from the tape recording:

"I went to Amravati in Maharashtra. At the church there I found a friend who I later met again in the hotel. My friend told me I should make a grave as the Bible tells us to do. I then went from the small church, which is not that nice, to the large church, where the Bible was lying. My friend told me to come in but I remained outside and wanted to go and eat. While I was eating the waiter told me I should leave my friend because he was after my money. I felt intimidated by this because my trust in him was destroyed. I went devotedly to Benares to a temple. Here I made my mother my wife for one night. That was in Muharram. You see, my wife who was my wife had left me. I didn't like that. And gradually my body turned cold-cold-cold. And then I was done for. Then I went to the *dargah* of Haji Abdul Rahman in Maharashtra and went inside. I sat down in front of this shrine. With that I saw Muhammad Mustafa Salela Salam in Arabistan and this Mecca and Medina and entered into *hajri* for Haji Abdul Rahman. A woman came and entered into *hajri* and had dreams. And I said to Haji Abdul Rahman that I oughtn't really to see these riches and Medina. I don't need such riches and don't like Medina. No, I don't want to see these riches, but the Haji said: `You have to see it, you must see it,' and then I began to see women's genitals everywhere and the Haji's wife pushed herself in front of him, and, you know, that's my house and my wife's there, God have mercy on me, and, you know, I then slept with my sister and then with my mother who had been my mother for many years. No, I cannot claim to be a man of honour because you can only become honourable through the Koran and through prayer." And then he added: "And through nothing else."

He paused briefly, took a deep breath, threw his arms with the chains up in the air, took another deep breath and continued in his sing-song voice: "Then you achieve the natural state of grace, and once there I said to my wife: we are one." He paused again and then said: "I led an easy life... at the cost of the women..., and then my wife went to Haji Abdul Rahman with the children and said that I was now superfluous. But then he granted her justice. But what is justice under Islam, the one between brothers and sisters or the one between the castes and religions?" His gaze turned inwards: "Allah is infinite and so is his prophet," he said, and: "Coming from the world of Islam we reached the world of medicine, of the moon and rockets." He slumped down and fell silent, and remained that way for so long that we felt he had nothing more to say and began to leave — he seemed that unwilling to converse.

But suddenly he reared up, wrung his chained hands and said in a loud, insistent voice, almost as if holding an address: "A woman who reads the Koran, I stuck my penis into the mouth of a woman like that at her request. Afterwards she washed herself, purified herself and read prayers. She is my love, and love is holy. Love is also something. In God's name it is quite certainly something." Then he shouted: "I shall die now. My funeral shall be in London. My funeral will be given a 21-gun salute. My body is to be transported from Delhi to London and flowers are to scattered over it both here and there. And the world will be shut down for three whole days, but India for just one day. My friends will attend my funeral. I am speaking quite sincerely," he shouted, "in my eyes I see nothing but innocence, everywhere."

Two days later, while he was promenading calmly, like many others, around the courtyard, he told Vikram Nath that he thought he was mad and should go to an asylum.

The psychotherapist who was visiting us at the time examined the man. He told us that he was suffering from a psychosis. The word psychosis was also used for the other two cases, the fourteen year-old boy and the "sword-dancer". In the third case the "exodus from the world" could be clearly sensed in his every sentence. His wife is no longer there. The relationship between man and wife has been destroyed. Sex takes place at impossible locations with impossible partners, such as his mother or a pious woman who reads the Koran. He is not "of this world", he wants to die, and while the world is supposed to shut down for three days he wants to have himself buried to a gun salute. He had literally spat out what he thinks of this world. We kept seeing him, sitting calmly or walking to and fro. And a single question from us brought his world tumbling down: "If you ask me", he said, "I must tell you I don't really know a thing about Islam". His world of love, of faith, hope and charity has been dashed by and during his life. A psychosis? Doubtless an affliction, but one chosen by a person who wishes to turn his back on everything.

The men or boys who are brought to Mira Datar act fundamentally differently to the women. The male clients, or patients rather, do not enter *hajri*. They do not tell of some other plane of reality inhabited by *ballas* and *bhuts*. No demon or demoness speaks from them. They appear rather to produce a collage of realities, an amalgam of the world in which they live and in which they flounder.

Against this the women let another speak, an evil, cruel and cunning spirit. They produce complete stories, spread out entire life histories before us. The men let us peer though a kaleidoscope of sex, power, betrayal and abandonment. While the voices that the women give voice to tell a story, the men allow an insight into their wounds and disfigurement. The reality that they reveal is dashed and irreparable.

We only met a few men during all the years I visited the tomb who said that they had been in *hajri*. One had taken Tajinder as his example and told everyone: "My hair in which the *balla* was living has been cut off and is now lying in the *mujawars'* office."

Nobody paid any attention to him, even though he kept returning to it. A tale of bewitchment always involves two aims: that of the conjurer and his client to destroy the victim, and that of the victim to discover and expose the magic and liberate herself from it. The women use this path as a possibility for increasing their freedom to move and for extending their range of action, for this is very tightly circumscribed in Hindu and Muslim India. Male pilgrims evidently do not need to enter this path or use it for their strategic ends, so *hajri* remains largely a mode of expression for women, a "language" for those closed and locked in by their culture. What did Mazar say to me: "Women are more easily possessed by evil spirits, for they are in any case always *napak*."

On the other hand, these men, who are so unapproachable in their so-called psychoses, are undergoing a phase of deep-rooted crisis. They see their lives as destroyed and mutilated, and withdraw from them.

Consequently we asked the one and only man who said that he entered *hajri* to tell us his story, to which he obliged at once. His is a "feminine" story. At first he was compelled by physical complaints to visit the doctor. He had suffered from diarrhoea, frequent diarrhoea over the years, and although the doctors had been unable to find any physical causes, they had nevertheless given him "four hundred injections" which had cost him his all he had. In the end another technique was able to help him: *hajri*! His two paternal uncles had put out a bewitchment contract because he had taken some of their land. The demon that was ordered to enter his body was meant to destroy him. While he told us his story a rosary slipped all the while back and forth between his fingers. By entering *hajri* he discovered the cause of his illness, the magic. He underwent the cure at Datar's court, as he put it, and drank the water that had circled seven times around the tomb, wore an amulet from the saint and inhaled incense. He remained for hours on end seated in prayer in the courtyard. But he did not have to undergo any punishments like the ones we encountered in the women's cures.

And then he had a dream. It told him of a small *dargah* which he was to erect for Mira Datar in his village, for he saw a treasure trove of silver and gold in his field. He saw himself in his dream sleeping before this temple, from which a scent of incense emanated, and as he awoke he saw the green roof of the temple. In his dream he entered the temple and lying there curled up beneath magnificent shrouds was the sleeping saint, who was the size of a child.

He told this dream to Siraj Myan, his *mujawar*, whom he asked to accompany him and help dig up the treasure in his field and share it with him. But Siraj Myan adhered to the rules. He told the man that he could only travel with him if he, too, had a corresponding dream containing a *hukm*, an order. Siraj Myan dreamt:

He saw a young, fair-skinned and simply clad horseman approaching him.[5] At the same time the pilgrim was in *hajri* in the inner courtyard. The horseman said to the *mujawar*, "Your pilgrim will remain here another twenty-one days, his *balla* will be completely extinguished, and then he will depart."

The man had to dig out his treasure on his own because the *mujawar's* dream had not indicated any travel. This concluded the story of the man who had freed himself from his spell through *hajri* and wanted to become a treasure-seeker, thus turning it into a "male" story after all.

It is clear then that the pilgrims can be divided into very specific groups. On the one hand there are the women who make stories with their demons and she-demons — the possessed women of the Mira Datar Dargah. Then there are the men of all age groups whose world has collapsed and who have become psychotic. And then there are the pilgrims who flood into the inner courtyard, bringing their worldly, physical and mental problems to the shrine, and who want to receive the saint's blessing, to read the Koran or simply need to be near the *karamat* and to fill themselves with the saint's "good energy".

NOTES

1. Basu (1993) describes a visit to the *sidi* fakirs during the *urs* of Mira Datar, in which she gives a detailed description of the *Sidis'* role as fakirs.
2. For *chillas* see notes 11 (ch. 3) and 11, as well as Chapter III.
3. Menstruating women and women who have just given birth are excluded from religious acts in almost all parts of the world. This can be found in Hinduism, Islam, Judaism, in various forms of Christianity and even in cultures without writing, such as among the Baruyas in New Guinea.
4. The term "therapy management group" was coined by John Janzen in his work *The Quest for Therapy in Lower Zaire*, (Berkeley, University of California Press, 1978). It refers to that group of people who reach all relevant decisions from the beginning of an illness to the end, and thus determine its course. As such the healers are not part of this group. However, the *mujawars* have such a strong influence on family decisions that they can be referred to as *therapy managers* with impunity.
5. Pictures of saints always show fair-skinned faces. A fair skin stands for pure, noble and elect. It was the fair skin of the rider in the dream that revealed his identity to the dreamer.

Chapter 7

The Women, their Psychology and Possession

What kept fascinating me and my friends and fellow travellers at the tomb of Mira Datar was the way that exceptional states of consciousness were handled in public. The *public* display of the state of possession in trance drew us as if by magic and fascinated us. During my work at the tomb I tried to recall when our culture had lost what I was witnessing here. My associations were with "hysterical women" and "witch-hunts". Nothing else wanted to enter my mind when I attempted to think about *our* history.

Generally we think of other cultures when we hear the terms trance, possession or exceptional states of consciousness, because "that's obvious!" We are reminded of oracular priests in Tibet or *Candomblé* in Brazil or *Voodoo* in Haiti. Perhaps on occasion of the Zar cult in east Africa. And some may be reminded of the Balinese art of trance after having read Margaret Mead's books, or simply because they have travelled there.

Perhaps some will even recall the European example of Soeur Jeanne des Anges of Loudon, who became renowned throughout the whole of France as a result of her cleverly staged possession by the Devil — so clever that not she, but Urbain Grandier, the local priest, was burned at the stake. Soeur Jeanne des Anges was undoubtedly full of cunning, and not without reason did Aldous Huxley write a book on her. But our thoughts about trance, as an everyday and public phenomenon, always lead us initially to foreign parts.

The ethnographic discourse on trance began during the middle of this century. Western observers to Africa were drawn by their fascination for the topic to Haiti, Bali and India, where they found something that no longer exists here, which has been excluded from society and forced to lead a shadowy existence in the (literary) underground. The names Hîlderlin, Dostojevsky and Artaud come to mind here. And before that Shakespeare, Cervantes and, even further in the past, Hieronymous Bosch, who also commemorated "the great prestige of madness" as Foucault, who describes its decline, has put it.

"Where's my fool?" complains King Lear when beset by early childhood desires, for the words of a fool are better nourishment than the milk of even the best wet-nurse.

Michael Foucault, the renowned theorist on exclusion and power, has described the journey undertaken by madness, or the "constant error", once left from our society in his acribic book *Madness and Civilisation*. The rise of Western society is a staging of the way the tragic, the savage, the structured error is erased from memory. It is also a staging of the parting. Parting from the dream, as Foucault says. And to he adds this the more disturbing severance when he speaks of the obstinate forms of regression — not merely in order to write down a chronicle of morals and tolerance, but also in order to show that the tragic severing of the happy world of sensual pleasure represent a border of the Occident and a source of its morality. Is it possible to find a culture with reason but without madness, Foucault asks, then adding that "... in our culture there can be no reason without madness, even if the rational knowledge that is gained from madness both reduces and disarms the latter *by giving it the fragile status of a pathological error.*"

The parting of the Orient and the Occident is similarly a product of the rationality that came into being in the West. The Orient, which is thought of as a wellspring, and is proffered to the colonialist reasoning of the Occident "and yet remains eternally inaccessible, .. remains the night of the beginning in which the Occident formed itself..." (Foucault,

1965,). Is that the origin of our fascination? The undisguised profession of a state of consciousness that has long since been assigned the status of a pathological error in our culture?

Let us recall briefly all that Teresa of Avila, who was "possessed by the Man of Sorrows", had to do during the period of the interior consolidation of power in Spain in order to establish that hers was a true, mystical path, and that she should *not* be mistaken for a crazed, possessed, or mad woman or for someone in league with the Devil. She was not declared a witch or denounced as a "hysterical woman": she became a saint.

Similarly the anorectic Katherine of Siena needed witnesses in order to proceed, protected, along her path. Pater Raimondo had to supervise the dietetic practices of this "wilful" mystic for the Vatican in order to exclude the possibility of devilish activities (Bell, 1985).

For the possessed were apprehended on two occasions in Europe: firstly during the sixteenth century by the Church and state, and secondly during the eighteenth and nineteenth centuries, when the Church wished to hear from the doctors, as indeed it came to hear from them, that such phenomena as ecstasy, inspiration, prophetism and inspiration by the holy ghost were simply the product of violent flushes and the heating of the humours (Foucault, 1965).

We even had to listen to these arguments at the tomb: it was the heat in the body that produced the mischief. Heat is dangerous in the body, in sexuality and in trance. When the *Sidi* fakirs or their women sing in trance at weddings, funfairs or during the *urs*, they must be given cooling substances such as cow milk, or "cooling" texts must be sung and the rhythm of the drums slowed down so that the women are not corrupted by the heat (Basu, 1993, p.166).

During the period of their segregation in Europe, madmen were either placed in specially designated hospitals, or they became famous. Up till around 1650, writes Foucault, "Western culture was curiously receptive" (1954) to madness and the prodigious. But this suddenly changed: the world of the mad became the world of the segregated. We know the story from

Foucault's book *Madness and Civilisation* (1965), in which he describes the changing ideologies behind the great internment.

Before the nineteenth century the perception of madness in Western society was very polymorphic. The fact that our era conceives of it under the term "illness" should not belie its original richness.

And the fact that psychology is unable to cope with madness also has its reasons: psychology was only first possible in our world once madness had already been mastered and excluded from the drama. Psychology falls silent and is quite unable to utter a word when confronted by the language (or screams) of a Nerval, Nietzsche or Artaud — a language that derives the meaning of *its* words from a freedom which the mere existence of "psychologists" guarantees will be sealed over by an oppressive forgetting and made inaccessible to humanity today (Foucault, 1965).

Hence the ethnographic discussion on trance, ecstasy and possession arose from a longing for what had been forgotten. And soon this longing was no longer to be stilled in the West.

Maya Deren, the New York actionist, underground film-maker and film-making ethnographer, became one of the first to express this longing in the west after seeing the films of Bateson and Mead on Balinese trance. In 1947 she went to Haiti in order to capture the ritual of voodoo by artistic means. She returned with six hours of exposed film, but without ever editing and using them. Instead she wrote a book entitled *The Divine Horsemen — Living Gods of Haiti*. In the foreword she refers to her inability to exploit the film material as an artistic failure. But what she is alluding to here is a deeper issue, one which every ethnographer must face: how is she to find her way back out of the ethnographic experience without foundering on the conflict between scientific concept and emotional abandon.

Is it possible to understand rituals of possession without personal belief or experience? It is generally considered that something has been understood when it can be translated into familiar categories and designated by specialised terms. Maya Deren's film material was worked posthumously into a one-hour version. Yet even this rudiment shows once again the inward-turned gaze of the dancer possessed by his god. The premises of scientific conduct demand distance to the subject. Maya Deren was unable to maintain this when confronted with the Haitian rituals, nor did she even wish to do so. She was torn out of her context in the truest sense of the word. Her art was bound to fail so long as she did not yield herself to the alien context posed to her by the Other. The great American scholar of religion and anthropology, Joseph Campbell, who was also fascinated by the inexplicable, wrote about Maya Deren in the foreword to her book: "Maya Deren went first to Haiti as an artist thinking to make a film in which Haitian dance would be a leading theme. But the manifestation of rapture that first fascinated and then seized her transported her beyond the bounds of any art she had ever known. She was open to the messages of that speechless deep, which is, indeed, the wellspring of all mysteries."

Maya Deren's work numbers among the classic attempts to understand, to grasp and to be moved by trance. Further important works come from the pen of Lorna Marshall.

Lorna Marshall filmed, described and danced 31 times the trance dance of the !Kung San. That was in the 1950s. The !Kung San call the spiritual energy which raises them above their everyday lives, *num*. *Num* is strong, and thus they also call it a "death thing" or a "struggle". *Num* is the power of the deity Gao Na. Every healer can receive it from him. During the healing dance of the !Kung San the num energy is all-prevailing. It burns within the fire of the dance; it emanates from the dance songs; it is inside the healers. It can be felt in the pit of the stomach, and it also has its seat at the base of the spine. When the *num* rises the dancer or healer enters *kia*. It is necessary to experience *kia* in order to be able to heal. It is a painful, dreaded experience. Katz asked the old healer Kinachau about it, and the man told him what it is like to experience *kia*.

"You dance, dance, dance, dance. The *num* lifts you up in your belly and lifts you in your back, and you start to shiver. *Num* makes you tremble; it's hot. Your eyes are open, but you don't look around; you hold your eyes still and look straight ahead. But when you get into *kia* you're looking around because you see everything, because you see what's troubling everybody. Rapid shallow breathing draws *num* up. What I do in my upper body with the breathing, I also do in my legs with the dancing. You don't stomp harder, you just keep steady. Then *num* enters every part of your body, right to the top of your feet and even your hair." (Katz, 1982)

The *num*, this "deadly thing", this vital energy from the Kalahari Desert which allows all who enter *kia* to see everything that makes people ill, this conceptualisation and use of the life and healing energy has reached us, first through the ethnographic discussion of the Other, and secondly by the awareness of the "alien world" that makes the Other comprehensible. Lorna Marshall and Richard Katz were not reduced to silence like Maya Deren who, instead of editing her film, was compelled to stage voodoo rituals and with that stage-manage herself. Instead of this, they reported on it.

But trance is still something that only exists for the Other, in "other parts". We Europeans are permitted to learn the use of ayahuasca, mescaline and psilocybin from *shamans* in the two American continents and thus discover exceptional states of consciousness, or learn trance dances from Africans and meditation techniques from Indians and Japanese. But at the same time our medical system gives us a psychiatry which, in its last but one "profession of faith", the DSM III-R (Diagnostic statistical manual III-Revised), has turned the clock back to the end of the last century, hoisted the flag of Kraepelin and excluded the Other (Young, 1991). And worse still: this psychiatry is being exported to Third World countries that are the first world in terms of mastering consciousness and all that is concerned with trance dances, trance and the recognition of illness through trance and visions.

Ethno-medical reports show however that although such psychiatric facilities are already being employed in Java, Africa and India, at the same time support continues to be sought in and provided by local healing traditions (Pfleiderer and Bichmann 1985). Let us recall the pilgrims and the sick in the inner courtyard of the tomb. Many of them were briefly exposed to the psychiatric institutions of their land. And many of them were brought to the inner courtyard because they were "hopeless cases".

While I sat in the inner courtyard of the tomb and watched young women like Subeida and Razia screaming and raging through the halls of the tomb, I kept asking myself about the *history of our bodies*. But no sooner did the question arise than it vanished again. I brushed it aside, like one of the bothersome flies at the tomb. The question of the history of the body in our own culture produced a feeling of physical discomfort in me. And the question of the history of the female body in our culture led me constantly and unwillingly to associations with "hysterical women" or "witch-hunts". The things that were happening at the tomb were for me uncanny in the truest sense of the word. And if I had given free rein to my associations or whole genealogies of associations, something very painful would have emerged.

Because every woman in the culture of central Europe "knows" on a level of physical perception how, during the last two to three hundred years, she has been made a "witch", a "hysteric", a "suffragette" and finally — as if she now wished physically to disappear — an "anorectic". She cannot forget the titles of such books as *Vom physiologischen Schwachsinn beim Weib* [= On Physiological Dementia in Women] (Moebius, 1900) or *Das Weib bei den Primitiven* [= Women among Primitive Peoples] (Reitzenstein, 1900), as well as the records of the witch trials from several centuries previously. Yet this knowledge, which in the final analysis can be reduced to a common conceptual denominator like "woman as illness" (Fischer-Homberger, 1979), is not "active" when a female anthropologist sets out to learn about the spaces occupied by women in other cultures. This knowledge is not part of her personal baggage. The body's memory does not remain silent, though, no more than does the collective unconscious. It sends signals along the pathways of our dreams or colours our perceptions. I described in Chapter V "The Female Anthropologist's Dream". The agents that attempted to disrupt the woman's ethnographic work at the shrine and who made her feel so uncertain were male. Where did this uncertainty come from?

The ideology of the tomb says that it is women who go into trance, and only rarely the men. Demons and she-demons speak from the women, and rarely from the men. "If our women are incautious when they attend to nature's call," said Mazar the *mujawar*, "a spirit will enter them — from below." No such thing is said about the men at the tomb. So it is a question of boundaries. The ideology of the tomb defines the boundaries of the women analogously to the Hindu or Muslim world picture in India, while the women overstep the boundary when they enter into trance. And they do this in public. But while they do this voices speak from them. Thus they undermine their social boundaries — "with the techniques of hysteria, as it were" (Braun, 1985, p.93). They are no longer people when they succumb to the trance and step onto the stage, rather they are woman plus demoness. And in this form they may speak. For their words "are... the (perhaps strongest) expression of *rebellion* against the destruction of their egos to take place on a collective level," writes Christina von Braun in her incomparable study on hysteria as a means of reversing the collective process of forgetting (Braun, 1985).

And then memory begins to function again.

Didn't my thoughts circle round another stage while writing this book, one that had been public in the most embarrassing way? The "saints" and "administrators" of this stage were also men. And the women were the puzzle, an inscrutable phenomenon which the men could not and would not grasp (Bernheimer and Kahane, 1985). It was this stage that became one of the bases of Freudian psychology: the stage of Charcot, the famous French psychiatrist who presented and treated "hysteric" women (and men) at the Salpetriére in Paris and to whom Freud briefly apprenticed himself.

Yes, I thought about Charcot's stage so much that I did not wish to picture it to myself for one single moment during my work at the tomb. If I had done so I would have become one of them, one of the possessed; with that I would have had to face the thousand year-old history of the demonising and colonising of woman: my history. Because no woman is able to escape Charcot's stage in this sense. And no woman plays the woman's role so perfectly as the hysteric. It is hysteria that causes so much confusion because "with its assistance woman is transformed ... into a myth" (Braun, 1985). Likewise the idiom of possession at the tomb transforms the women into a myth, and the two transformations have one thing in common:

It is not the woman *herself* who is speaking, it is a demon (at the tomb) or animal (in antiquity) who speaks from her. Both here and there it is the Devil in person who has to be placated. Above all in modern times, during which woman's knowledge of nature and plants and above all of healing has been taken away from her, *man* wanted to be safe in the "knowledge" that it was the Devil who was talking from a healing woman.

This animal that is supposed to reside in her has already been attributed to woman for some four thousand years. We come across it for the first time in ancient Egyptian medicine. The "Kahun Papyrus of 1900 BC and the Ebers Papyrus (around 1600 BC) both talk of 'women's complaints,' which were roughly expressed by paralysis or choking fits, and for which the doctors were unable to find any organic explanation" (Braun, 1985, p.34). These symptoms appear solely among women and not among men. The symptoms were diagnosed as "starvation" of the womb — as if this were some animal that had not been fed. The womb was thus a kind of animal that resided inside the woman's body, an animal that began restlessly to wander about when the womb remained unsatisfied. With that the animal had to be soothed, because it would cause choking fits if it wandered upwards and paralysis if it wandered downwards. It was lured downwards by pleasant fragrances which were used to fumigate the vagina, or by unpleasant odours which were introduced from above through the mouth. This concept of the animal in woman, of the womb as a foreign body, also reached Greece, where it became wide-spread. It can be found in Plato, as well as in

Hippocrates, who in his medical texts recommended a highly simple cure for calming the animal: marriage and pregnancy (Bernheimer, 1985, p.3). And Plato called the animal "a living being desirous of child-bearing, which grows 'recalcitrant' when it 'remains without fruit' for long." (Braun, 1983, p.35).

The women at the tomb have grasped "their history" when they open up their space during trance. With this they have also "sealed over" their history within the sub-continent's (two-fold) patriarchy.

But in our case the net has become increasingly tight, because parallel to the history of the development and decline of hysteria in Europe came the colonisation of the female body, or more precisely "the administration of the female interior from which the body politic must be produced" (Duden, 1987). This state colonisation of the uterus was performed by the "administrators" of medicine, who turned the womb into a vessel.

The decline of hysteria as a great myth *in* women's act of refusal has brought "recollection" to a standstill. It was this standstill that I became conscious of while talking to the women at the tomb. All of the stories at the tomb are "stories of bewitchment". At the beginning of almost every one is a bewitchment contract. And the menstrual blood that has "accidentally" landed in the food in order to rob the victim — male or female — forever of his senses.

I would likewise have been robbed of my senses if I had thought of the witch trials of the *Holy* Inquisition while noting down the tales of bewitchment I was told by the women (and men) at the tomb. While watching the bodies writhing in trance at the tomb, I might well have thought of those other tortured bodies which were accused at the witch trials of having slept with the Devil, simply because they had put themselves around some *datura* or other such substance right there where the body politic was supposed to be born. No, I was quite right not to think of Charcot's stage for hysterics or of the way the torture cages were put on display during the inquisition while I was working on the women' stage at the tomb.

The shutting down of the memory, of the collective

memory, "worked" during the personal ethnographic process which led to this study. Otherwise I would have been unable to rob the women's stage at the tomb of its history while writing my description. And Muhammadhusen also played his part when he confirmed to me that the women in trance were a phenomenon which had no history at the tomb. Yet the women at the tomb capture a space for themselves with their *hajri* play, one that they had lost when their bodies were buried alive twice over by the principle of patriarchy. The one principle is upheld by the Indian theory of society (*Dharmashastra*), which radically restricts woman's space. The other principle was brought to the women of India by the colonisation of their land and their bodies by the Europeans, above all the 19th-century British who came from the Victorian era of bodily alienation. This is the reason why I term it a "two-fold" patriarchy.

And yet the women fascinated us with their play. For they are full of cunning, these women.

The women at the tomb enter trance with a specific mental set and within a specific setting. Their everyday lives are reflected in both their experiences and their behaviour during trance. Mostly they induce trance by means of hyperventilation and the strong, indeed imperative notion that they are possessed by an evil spirit, and that they are stepping while in this impure state before the hallowed grave of a saint. They undergo a process of trance and interpretation, dream and interpretation, bodily perception and interpretation. They call this process healing or a cure. And it is their interpretation of the course of the process that produces the cure that has to be explained or declared as such to the outside world. Their trance, which they call *hajri*, meaning evil spirit possession, makes the possession manifest in sight and sound.

And everyone who goes to the court to be cured "wants" just one thing: that the spirits leave their body, their head and their life. And yet: the spirits speak out loud from them and say that they want to remain, don't want to budge, will spit back.

We invited the women to make drawings, asking them:

"What do you see when you are in trance?"

Razia drew flowers, just flowers, over and over again. And she said: "That's what I see when I'm in trance, flowers...."

Razia couldn't have found a better weapon against the annihilation of her ego than flowers.

Outlook

It is our last evening in Unava. Vikram Nath and I am sitting and eating at Sardarji's. We have spent a number of weeks during each of the last five years listening to the *mujawars* and the possessed women. Their stories are documented by an impressive number of tapes, notebooks and colour slides. We have had hundreds of questionnaires filled out with case histories, personal disaster and cures. We have had over fifty *mujawars* fill out questionnaires on themselves. We have amassed file upon file of historical documents concerning the tomb and, either jointly or singularly, have given talks and lectures and written articles on the tomb. We finally decide on this evening that we have completed our study: *hukm*. We had found answers to all of our questions, those that we brought with us and those that we discovered there. We are sitting with Sardarji in the midst of the joint history of our research that I have described in this book.

"What shall we do next?" we ask ourselves over lentils with ginger, spinach with cheese and all of the other delicacies of the Punjabi cuisine.

"Let's do a study on the *hijras*!" I suggest, and think with a thrill of the unkempt women at the temple of the goddess Bahuchara who are not what they seemed. "No one has been there yet."

"Why do you keep on having to scouring the most perverse fringes of our society?" asks Vikram Nath, who suggests that we visit the most perverse temple that a Westerner could even imagine in order that I lose my taste for such topics.

I protest, saying with feigned objectivity: "Do you think it was perverse to write about your Hindi films, which lure millions of hungry stomachs into the cinemas each evening?"

"Yes," says Vikram Nath, and he closes the subject.

But he has an idea that awakens my curiosity.

"Let's travel tomorrow or the day after to Bikaner. That's right at the top of north-west Rajasthan. You'll enjoy that because you can only reach it by the *chhoti* line, the narrow gauge railway."

"And what are we going to do there?" I ask, worried, because Vikram Nath sounds so pedagogic.

"We'll visit the most perverse temple you can imagine. We can stay with some friends of mine, don't worry, it'll all work out," he reassures me.

"I've only four days left, are you sure we can manage it in that time?"

"I just mean one temple and not a thousand and one. Of course we'll manage it. From there you can return to Delhi on the *chhoti* line," he replies with a grin, "and I'll travel back home to Mumbai. Where's the problem?"

I agree. We spend a whole day packing our documents and momentoes and the day after take the train to Bikaner. We arrive there unwashed, hungry and thirsty after a night in the train. Our teeth grate from the soot and the dust of the narrow gauge railway. Vikram Nath had notified two of his friends that we are coming, and they are waiting for us at the platform. One of them is a university professor, the other a *vaidya*, a doctor specialised in ayurvedic medicine. We are put up in the latter's beautiful house. Downstairs is the doctor's surgery, which faces on to the inner courtyard where he has his herb garden. Upstairs are the rooms inhabited by his family. Bikaner is a desert town with one or more princely palaces and a hot, dry climate. It is a great relief to rest in the cool of the house among the plants.

"What do you want to do this afternoon?" our host inquires.

"We're driving to the poet's temple at Deshmok," Vikram Nath replies without first waiting to listen to me.

We arrange to meet up in the early afternoon. Our hosts promise that they will have found a car for us by then.

That afternoon the car is standing before the door, as arranged. We get inside, Vikram Nath, his two friends and myself, and make the thirty-minute journey through the desert to Deshmok. A village looms up. We stop at a largish square and get out.

"My God, Vikram Nath, look over there on the temple wall, it's teeming with rats," I call.

But Vikram Nath is not alarmed by my observation. He does not even stop to look. Instead he looks at me with the most cryptic smile he can muster during the betel season, and says:

"That's what we talked about, you're now going to see one of the most perverse temples there is, look — it's just as I promised."

The three men walk over to the temple, grinning, and invite me to accompany them. "This is the poet's temple of Deshmok," they say, then adding mischievously: "It's not yet been discovered by tourists." I am incredibly curious but simultaneously I have a creepy feeling. I follow them. As at every temple in India one has to take off one's shoes at the entrance. I have some difficulty in doing what is expected of me as a result of the numerous rats that are roaming around. I slowly slip off my shoes and place them with the others.

"You must just watch out for one thing," my companions tell me, "no one may tread on any of the rats of Deshmok because they are holy."

"Does that mean that there are also rats inside the temple?" I ask, intimidated.

"Yes," says Vikram Nath, "come on, we're going inside."

While he says this our host takes me by the hand and leads me through the door of the temple into the courtyard. The ground here is a living carpet of rats which are busily attending to their daily affairs, undisturbed. I hold my bag at ankle height so that I can ward them off, to one side at least. But on the other side they are free to scrabble over my and indeed all of our feet, which they do.

We approach the next door which leads into the temple. Here the number of rats increases to such an extent that we are up to our calfs in rats, who don't pay the slightest heed to the newcomers. We continue our way to the inner sanctum, wading up to our knees in rats as if through a river. We work our way forward to the altar, and the rats scamper in the same direction. What can they be after there? How is the *puja,* the ceremony of worship performed here?

On closer inspection we discover a mound of sugar which is offered to the holy rats as food. The things they offer in temples, I reflect. And to whom? My goodness. Simply nothing is impossible in India. So this is the poet's temple of Deshmok!

The rats teem over the mound of sugar inside the temple and over all of the side altars. Rats. Thousands upon thousands of rats.

My host is still holding on tight to my hand. The stench of rats creates a feeling of anxiety in me. We push our way forward to the altar and make our offering: of course, I recall, we had bought a small bag of sugar from a tradesman at the entrance. And then we make our way back out and across the courtyard, and finally to the exit. Back on the road outside the rats that are scurrying along the walls seem to be nothing more than a handful of isolated individuals that I scarcely notice.

"What did you mean by poet's temple?" I ask, still slightly out of breath after concentrating myself so long against my rising nausea and revulsion. Our host replies:

"There used to be a poet at the Royal court whose job was to entertain the King. One day the poet, whom the King deeply admired, suddenly died and the King was plunged into grief at the loss. The King went one last time to the bed of his beloved friend, who was to be cremated the next day, and asked: 'What can I do for you?' Suddenly a rat appeared on the poet's head, where it stopped and gazed intently at the King. The King let it carry on and that night he had a dream:

"During this dream the departed poet spoke to him, saying: 'In my next life I shall be a rat, and in the manner of rats, I will help to ensure that no rubbish accumulates in the palace. Please bestow your grace on the rats.'

"The King reported this to his subjects and ordered his master-builder to erect a temple in which rats would be worshipped and fed. And that's what you've just seen."

"So that's why it's called the poet's temple and not the rat temple!" I exclaimed, "You really took me for a ride with the way you referred to it!"

"We had to, after all I didn't want us to work on any more perversities. So I showed you one of the most perverse temples in the whole of Hindu India..."

We burst into liberating laughter. No, I certainly would never want to work here, Vikram Nath could be assured of that. But why on earth did he tell me in this way? India, an iconic culture? Yes, doubtless, and a culture of sight and sights.

Vikram and I worked together on a number of projects over the following years, but these no longer belonged, as Vikram Nath expected from an European anthropologist, to the "interspaces".

Glossary

Ambica	Indian mother goddess
arti	worship before an image of God using an oil lamp
asar ki namaz	evening prayer, prayers at five o'-clock
Ashraf	caste term among the Muslims
atman	soul
Babo Ind	local deity who can be traced back to the Vedic god Indra
Bahuchara	a goddess
bal(l)a	evil spirit, synonym for *bhut*
balian	Balinese healer
bapu	familiar term of address
barakat	dispensation of grace, blessing, holiness
bhajan	hymn of praise
bhakta	worshipper of a personal God, mystic
bhakti	(mystic) worship of God
Bhangi	sweeper, unclean caste
Bhil	ethnic group in northern India
bhut	evil spirit
bhutani	female, evil spirit
bhopas	specialist in possession, trance healer
Brahmin	member of the highest Hindu caste, priest
burka	a loose black gown that cloaks the entire body, worn by Muslim women
Chaitra	month of April
chalu chillai	ribbon handed to a person when they are discharged

chandra ma	a name for the moon
chapatti	a thin, flat loaf of unleavened wheat flour
chauk	place, locality
chilla	memorial shrine
Chishti	Muslim order
chhoti	small
churäl	a female spirit
churidar	loose breeches
dadi	father's mother
dadima	father's mother
dakhol	dance performed by a group of fakirs
dammal	dance, drum rhythm of the Sidi
danriya	specialist in possession in the Himalayas
darbar	court
dargah	place of pilgrimage, tomb of a Muslim saint
darzi	tailor
Datar	proper name
devi	goddess (generic)
Dharmashastra	classical teachings of the Hindus
dhol	large drum
dhoti	loin cloth, rural dress for men
dosas	originally: an error, but nowadays: bodily fluids
dupatta	veil combined with salwar-kamiz
ekveni	with a plait
fakir	fakir
farishta	angel
fatiha	1st Koran sura
Ganesh(a)	the elephant-headed god
Gao Na	a god among the !Kung-San in the Kalahari desert, Africa
gaun	village
ghar	house
ghee	clarified butter
ghum hajri	trance performed in silence
ghusl	ritual washing of the dead
gilaf	shroud
Golu	a god in the Himalayas

Goraknath	the same as Golu
Goril	the same as Golu
gotra	line of descent
gunas	means spirit (sattwa), passion (*rajas*), physical mass, sloth (*tamas*) or the human characteristics
gupta roga	mysterious illness
gurz	iron spike
Hadkair	a goddess
Haji	pilgrim to Mecca
hajiri ata	trance comes
hajri	trance
Halapati	a goddess
haldi	turmeric
Hanuman	monkey god from the *Ramayana*
Harai	a goddess
hijra	eunuchs
Hindustani	the language of northern India
Holi	spring festival among the Hindus, held at full moon in March
hukm	advice, directions
jadu	magic
jadugar	magician
jagar	vigil, shamanic ritual during the night in northern India
jagar khelna	to perform a therapeutic, shamanistic ritual
jagriya	singer during the jagar
Jain	member of the like-named religion
jaise	"just like..."
Jati	caste group
ji	suffix attached to a name as a term of respect
jinn	Muslim spirit
jinnat	Muslim spirit
jeera	cumin
kabrstan	Muslim cemetery
kapha	mucus, quality of same in ayurvedic medicine
karamat	ability to perform miracles
Katolia Rajputs	ethnic group

khanqah	Muslim hospice
kia	trance and ecstasy among the !Kung-San in the Kalahari, Africa
Kshatriyia	the warrior or land-owner caste
larkilog	the people from the bride's side
lingam	the penis of the god Shiva, which is venerated by Hindus
loa	spirit
loban	incense
Lohar	blacksmith
Mahakali	a goddess
Mahisa	buffalo demon
maika	parental home from the viewpoint of married Hindu women
mazzar sharif	sacred grave
mama	mother's brother
mamu-dargah	grave of the mother's brother
Mehendi	name of the king who slayed Mira Datar
Meghwal	low-caste group in north-west India
mela	festival, market
mehndi	a cooling dye
Mira	name of the saint
miti	sweet-tasting
mori	sewage
mujawar mudjavir	shrine attendant
murid	follower of a saint
murshid	spiritual leader
nagarkhana	drum house
nai	hair-dresser
napak	impure
ngoma	dance among the Sidis
nissandar	flag-bearer
Num	life energy among the !Kung-San, Kalahari, Africa
pagal	crazy
pak	pure
palit	spirit

pan	betel leaf preparation for chewing
paramparah	tradition
Parsis	a minority group who follow Zarathustra and mainly belong to the upper classes
Parvati	a goddess
pati dev	divine husband
Phalgun	the month of March
pir	a Muslim saint
pirzade	successor to a saint
pithi	turmeric paste
pitta	bile, quality of bile in ayurvedic medicine
pitu	spirit
prakrti	nature
prana	breath
prasad	divine food
puja	worship, reverential observance
pujari	temple attendant
purnima ka vrat	fast during the period of the full moon
purusha	the male principle
Rajput	landowner caste of Rajasthan
Ram Deo Pir	a saint
Rama	an incarnation of Vishnu, husband of Sita
randi	a female spirit
Rathva	ethnic group
Ravana	a deity, seducer and abducter of Sita
rawalia	fakir group
roga	sickness
sadar khalifa	chief of a fakir group
sadhu	ascetic or mendicant
sajjadanishin	chief of a sacred shrine
salwar	trousers
Samkhya	philosophical orientation
sandal-mujawar	shrine attendant who performs the ceremony during the urs
sardar	chief, leader
sardarji	term of address for a Sikh
sari	Indian woman's chief garment or dress
sas	a wife's mother-in-law

sasural	the home of the parents-in-law
sati	voluntary self-immolation on a funeral pyre by women, term for those who have committed this
sawwali	pilgrim at a tomb
seer	a unit of weight, approximately 2 pounds
Sem	a god
shadi	wedding
shahidana	martyrdom
shehnai	a kind of oboe
Shudras	the handworker caste
Sidis	ethnic group originating from Africa
Sita	a goddess from the Hindu epos the Ramayana
shaytan	Satan
Shiva	a supreme Hindu god
Suhrawardi	Sufi order
sulli	gallows, death
Sura	a chapter of the Koran
surya	sun
ta'widh	amulet
tabla	drum
Tadvi	ethnic group
tapas	heat
thali	plate, tray
triveni	a triple plait
umma	community of the faithful
urad	mung bean
Urdu	language spoken by south-Asian Muslims; also termed Hindustani
urs	the annual celebrations of the saint
Urs Sharif	the annual celebrations of the saint
vata	quality of wind in ayurvedic medicine
Vishnu	a supreme Hindu god

MIRA DATAR DARGAH AT UNAVA, GUJARAT

Latrine = latrines
Haupteingang = main entrance
Hof für psychotische Männer = court for psychotic men
Wassertank = water tank
Moschee = mosque
Läden = shops
Büros der Mujawars = offices of the *mujawars*
Waage = scales
Eingang = entrance
Baum = tree
Massen Quarteire = mass quarters
Gräber der Verwandten = relatives' graves
Silberzaun = silver fence
Grab = tomb
Nimbaum = neem tree
Männerhof = men's compound
Königskopf = king's head
Silberwand = silver wall
Gräber = graves
Fraunehof = women's compound
Unterkünfte = lodgings
Nebeneingang = side entrance
Kuppel der Dadima = Dome of Dadima
Friedhof = cemetry
Strasse nach Ahmedabad = road to Ahmedabad

Bibliography

Ahmad, Imtiaz, (ed.), 1981. Ritual and Religion among Muslims in India, New Delhi: Manohar.

Asch, Timothy and Linda O'Connor, 1986. Jero Tapakan. A Balian Spirit Medium, (film).

Basu, Helene, 1993. Fakire, Tänzer und Narren, Muslimische Heiligenverehrung bei den Sidi im nordwestlichen India, Dissertation, Berlin: Fachbereich Philosophie und Sozialwissenschaften.

Becker-Pfleiderer, Beatrix and Virchand Dharamsey, 1978. "Merkmale traditionellen Heilens in Gujarat", Internationales Asien Forum, 9, pp. 59–68, 192.

Bell, Rudolph, 1985. Holy Anorexia, Chicago: University of Chicago Press.

Bernheimer, Charles and Claire Kahane, (eds.), 1985. In Dora's Case. Freud-Hysteria-Feminism, New York, Columbia University Press.

Bernheimer, Charles, 1985. Introduction to Bernheimer, Charles and Claire Kahane (ibid.), pp. 1–18.

Bourguignon, Erika, 1976. Possession, San Francisco: Chandler and Sharp.

Braun, Christina von, 1985. Nicht ich, Frankfurt: Neue Kritik, p. 73, 75.

Currie, P. M, 1989. The Shrine and the Cult of Mu'in al-din Chishti of Ajmer, Oxford: Oxford University Press.

Das, G.N, 1991. Couplets from Kabir, New Delhi: Motilal Banarsidass Publisher.

De Certeau, Michel, 1980. La possession de Loudun, Paris: Gallimard.

Deren, Maya, 1953. Divine Horsemen. The Living Gods of Haiti, London: Thames and Hudson.

Duden, Barbara, 1987. Geschichte unter der Haut. Ein Eisenacher

Arzt und seine Patientinnen um 1730, Stuttgart, Klett-Cotta, p. 31.

Egnor, Margaret, 1983. "Death and Nurturance in Indian Systems of Healing", in *Social Science & Medicine* 17, No. 14, pp. 935–945.

Ende, Werner, 1991. "Mudjawir," in *Encyclopedia of Islam,* second edition. VII. Leiden, pp. 293–294.

Fischer, Eberhard, Jyotindra Jain and Haku Shah, 1982. Tempeltücher für die Muttergöttinnen in India. Zurich, Museum Rietberg, p. 82.

Fischer-Homberger, Esther, 1979. "Krankheit Frau, aus der Geschichte der Menstruation in ihrem Aspekt als Zeichen eines Fehlers", in Fischer-Homberger, (ed.), Krankheit Frau. Frankfurt: Suhrkamp, pp. 49–84.

Foucault, Michel, 1965. *Madness and Civilisation.* New York: Random House, p. 10.

Gaborieau, Marc, 1986. "Les ordres mystiques dans le sous-continent India. Un point de vue ethnologique", in Popovic, A. and G. Feinstein, Les ordres mystiques dans l'Islam, Paris: Editions de EHESS, p. 117.

Gazeteer of India/Gujarat State, 1975. Mehsana District: Government of Gujarat.

Grof, Stanislav, 1988. The Adventure of Self-Discovery, Albany: New York State University Press.

Helman, Cecil, 1987. "Heart Disease and the Cultural Construction of Time, The Type A Behaviour Pattern as Western Culture-bound Syndrome", *Social Science and Medicine,* 25, pp. 967–979.

Hiltbeitel, Alf, 1981. "Draupadi's Hair", in Autour de la Déèsse Hindou, M. Biardeau (ed.). Paris: Editions de EHESS, pp. 179–215.

Huxley, Aldous, 1952. *The Devils of Loudon,* London: Chatto and Windus.

Jain, Jyotindra, 1984. *Painted Myths of Creation,* New Delhi: Lalit Kala Akademi, p. 6.

Janzen, John, 1978. *The Quest for Therapy in Lower Zaire,* Berkeley: University of California Press.

Jeffery, Patricia, 1979. *Frogs in a Well, Indian Women in Purdah,* London: Zed Press.

Jeffery, Patricia, 1981. "Creating a Scene, the Disruption of Ceremonial in a Sufi shrine," in I. Ahmad 1981, pp. 162–194, in: Ritual and Religion among Muslims in India. Delhi: Manohar Book Service.

Kakar, Sudhir, 1978. *The Inner World,* Delhi: Oxford University Press.

Kapferer, Bruce, 1983. *The Celebration of Demons. Exorcism and the Aesthetics of Healing in Sri Lanka,* Bloomington: Indiana University Press.

Katz, Richard, 1982. *Boiling Energy,* Cambridge Mass., Harvard University Press, p. 42.

Latour, Bruno and Steve Wolgar, 1979. *Laboratory Life, The Social Construction of Scientific Facts,* Beverly Hills, California: Sage.

Lawrence, Bruce, 1978. Notes from a Distant Flute, the extant literature of the pre-Mughal Indian Sufism, Teheran: Imperial Academy of Philosophy.

Leiris, Michel, 1958. La possession et les aspects théatraux chez les Ethiopiens de Gondar, Paris: Plon.

Luig, Ute, 1990. "Körpermetaphorik, Sexualität und Macht der Frauen", in I. Lenz and U. Luig, (eds.), Frauenmacht ohne Herrschaft, Berlin: Orlandaverlag, pp. 255–279.

Marshall, Lorna, 1969. "The Medicine Dance of the !Kung Bushmen", in Africa, 39, pp. 347–381.

Michaels, Axel, 1986. *Gesellschaft und Ritual in India,* Frankfurt: Neue Kritik.

Mies, Maria, 1985. Indische Frauen zwischen Unterdrückung und Befreiung, Frankfurt: Syndikat.

Möbius, Paul Julius, Über den physiologischen Schwachseinn des Weibes. In: Sammlung zwangloser Abhandlungen aus dem Gebiete der Nerven- und Geisteskrankheiten, III Band, Heft 3, Halle : 1900.

Moffat, Michael, 1979. *An Untouchable Community in South India,* Princeton: Princeton University Press.

Nanda, Serena, 1990. *Neither Man nor Woman. The Hijras of India,* Belmont: Wadsworth Publishing Company.

Nawab All and Charles Norman Seddon, 1928. *Mirat-i-Ahmadi Supplement* (translated from the Persian by Ali Muhammad Khan), Baroda: Oriental Institute.

O'Flaherty, Wendy D, 1980. *Women, Androgynes, and Other Mythical Beasts,* Chicago: University of Chicago Press.

Obeyesekere, Gananath, 1981. *Medusa's Hair,* Chicago: Chicago University Press.

Obeyesekere, Gananath, 1985. "Depression, Buddhism, and the Work of Culture", in A. Kleinman and B. Good, *Depression and Culture,* University of S. California Press, pp. 134–152.

Pfleiderer, Beatrix, 1981. "Mira Datar Dargah, the Psychiatry of a Muslimshrine", in I.Ahmad 1981, pp.195-234. in *Ritual and*

Religion among Muslims in India. Delhi: Manohar Book Service.

Pfleiderer, Beatrix, 1983a. "Words and Plants, A Concept of Ayurvedic Psychotherapy," *Sociologus*, 33, pp. 25–41.

Pfleiderer, Beatrix, 1983b. "Jagar, A Therapeutic Vigil in Kumaun" (together with L. Lutze), *South Asian Digest of Regional Writing* 8, pp. 99–118.

Pfleiderer, Beatrix, 1984. "Nicht Krankheit ist's, schon Zauber", Curare Sonderband 2, pp. 115–124.

Pfleiderer, Beatrix, 1987. "Fremde im Haus", in A. Kuntz and B. Pfleiderer, ed., *Fremdheit und Migration*, Berlin: Reimer.

Pfleiderer, Beatrix, 1991. "Inszenierung des hinduistischen Familienmodells als Regelspiel der Frau", In, E. Berg et al, (eds.), *Ethnologie im Widerstreit*, MÅnchen, Trickster.

Pfleiderer, Beatrix and Wolfgang Bichmann, 1985. Krankheit und Kultur, Berlin: Reimer.

Pfleiderer, Beatrix and Lothar Lutze, 1985. *The Hindi Film, Agent and Reagent of Cultural Change*, Delhi: Manohar.

Pfleiderer, Beatrix and Gilles Bibeau, (eds.), 1991. "Anthropologies of Medicine" (*Curare* Sonderband), Vieweg: Wiesbaden.

Prescott, William, 1935. *The Conquest of Mexico*. London.

Reitzenstein, Carl Freiherr von. 1900. Das Weib bei den Primitiven. Duldthaus: Berlin.

Rollier, Franck, 1982. Murugmalla. Possession et Rituels Therapeutiques dans un Tombeau Musulman d'Inde du Sud, Etude Ethnopsychiatrique, La FacultÇ de Medicine de Bobigny.

Soeur Jeanne des Anges, *Autobiographie d'une hysterique possedee*, 1886. (eds), Drs Gabriel Legue and Gilles, de la Tourette, Paris.

Sen, Mala, 1991. *India's Bandit Queen, The True Story of Phulan Devi*, New Delhi: Indus, p. 215.

Stone, Hal and Sidra Winkelman, 1989. *Embracing Our Selves*, San Rafael, California: New World Library.

Young, Allen, 1991. "DSM-111 R and Kraepelin", in Beatrix Pfleiderer and Gilles Bibeau, (ibid.), 1991, pp. 175–181. Vieweg: Wiesbaden.

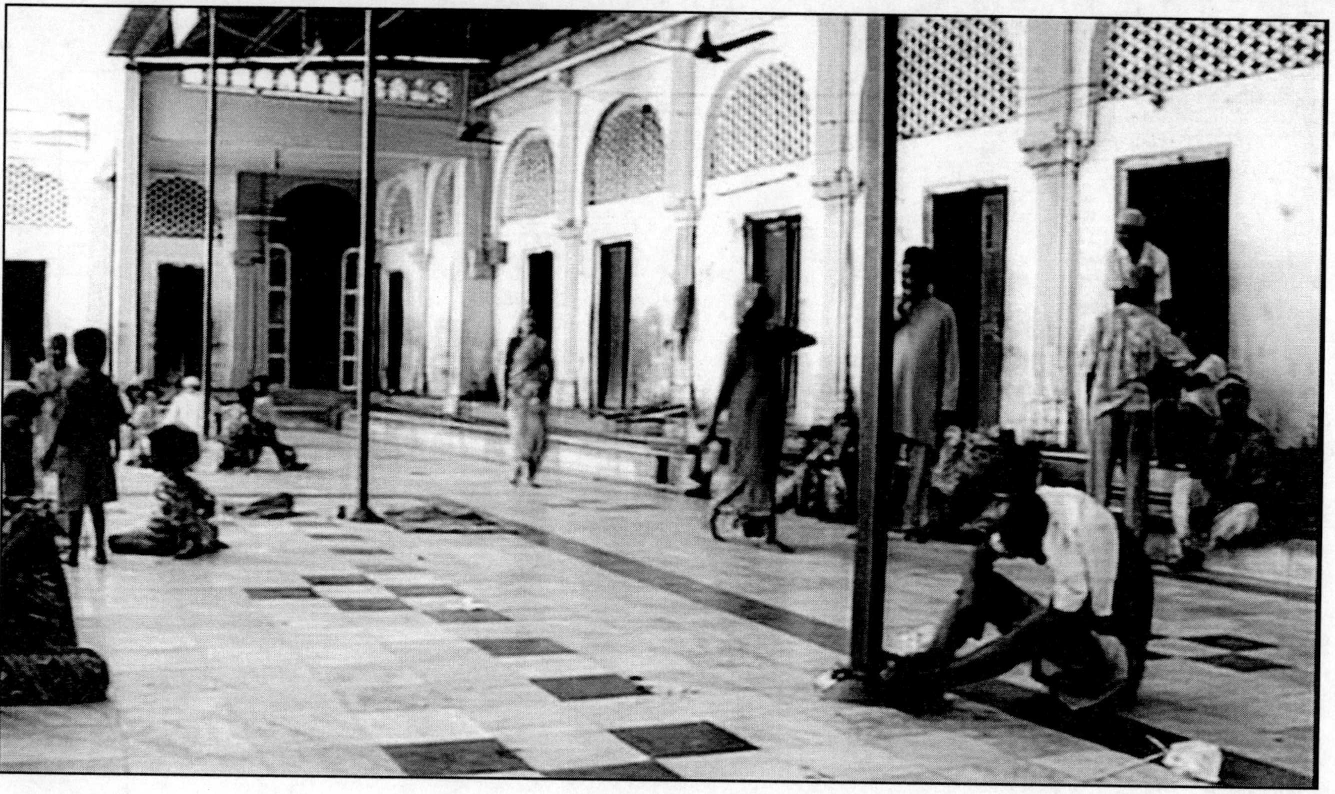

The Accommodations for the pilgrims

Groundplan of the Mira Datar tomb

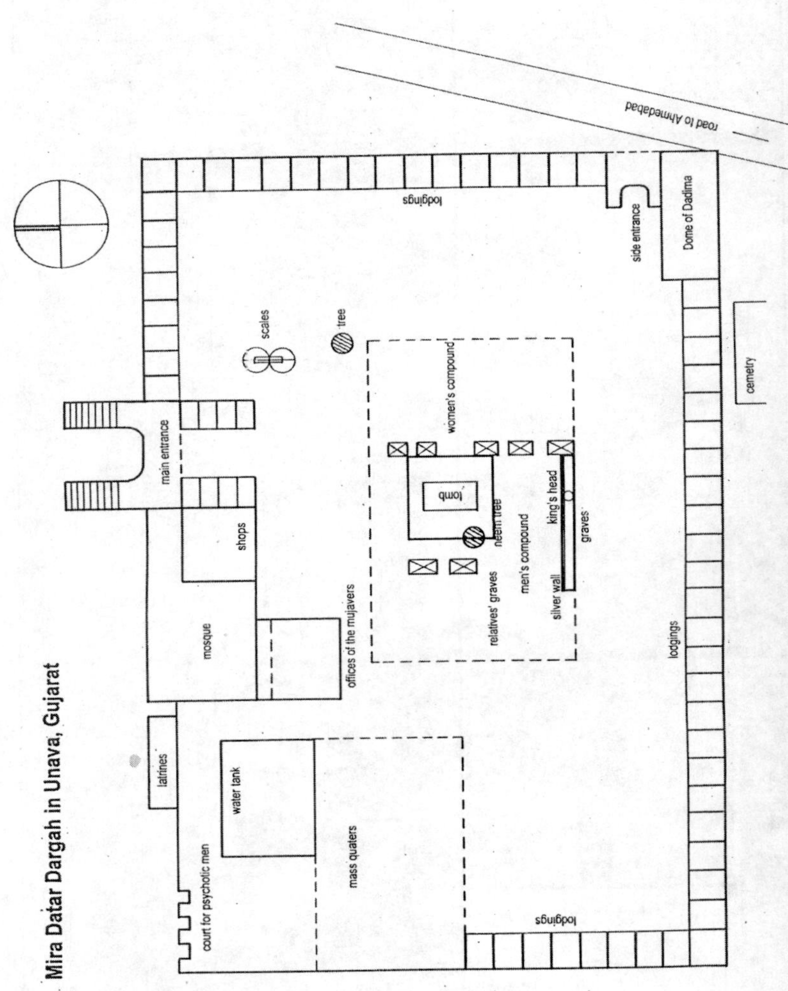

Mira Datar Dargah in Unava, Gujarat

Index